CITY LIFE

MICHAEL MORSE

Also by Michael Morse

Rescuing Providence
Rescue 1 Responding
Mr. Wilson Makes It Home

A POST HILL PRESS BOOK
ISBN: 978-1-68261-202-6
ISBN (eBook): 978-1-68261-014-5

City Life
© 2016 by Michael Morse
All Rights Reserved

Cover Design by Christian Bentulan

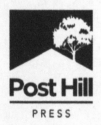

Post Hill Press
posthillpress.com

Published in the United States of America

For Lilyana Elizabeth, Kinsley Victoria, and Jaxon Chase

Here's to the future!

(Sorry, Jaxon, it's ladies before gentlemen in this house.)

CONTENTS

CONTENTS

FOREWORD

What kind of paramedic do I want to be?
How do I want to treat patients?
How do I want my patients and their families to remember me?
How can I avoid the burnout, cynicism, and hatred I see in other medics?

I found Michael Morse's blog, and first book, *Rescuing Providence*, soon after I became a paramedic. With each shift on the ambulance I was increasingly asking myself those questions.

I was working on-call and had a different partner on almost every shift. I had some great partners and some not so great partners. And we always had patients, many living on the very margins of society that either through their struggle with mental illness, addiction, incarceration or chronic illness brought out the best or the worst in us.

An unnecessary sternal rub on a drunk, an arm drop test on a seizing patient and high-speed driving and sharp turns felt more like patient assault than treatment.

Back at the station too many conversations tumbled downward to hate-filled, racial rants about the citizens of our response area. Looking back I suppose I could (and probably should of) taken a stand and confronted those medics.

Instead of joining the conversation or limply standing by I retreated into EMS books and blogs. Authors and EMS providers Michael Morse, Peter Canning, Kelly Grayson,

Thom Dick and Michael Perry taught me more than I had learned in medic school or from my preceptors. They were a much-needed counterbalance to what I was experiencing on duty.

I learned that it is OK to always give the patient the benefit of the doubt, that the best treatment might be a warm blanket and that if I didn't stand up for a patient no one would.

I also learned that the choices we make to be a part of EMS have consequences on our loved ones. Did I really need the overtime shift, side job teaching or second job at a different service?

Morse also showed me an outlet for the stress I was experiencing on the street. I needed an outlet that was safe for me, my wife and my young children. Like Morse I turned to writing, as well as exercise, to let go of the stress and not redirect it at my patients.

As you read *City Life* – a collection of patient encounters – don't mourn for Morse, look down at what he did or didn't do for his patients, or even judge the patients. Instead reflect on your own practice as a caregiver. What kind of paramedic, parent, spouse or friend do you want to be?

Greg Friese, MS, NRP
EMS1, editor-in-chief

INTRODUCTION

There comes a time when every one of us will need somebody. It is unavoidable. No matter how independent, isolated, or self-sufficient a person wishes to be, there is no escaping that fact. None of us can do it alone. Many have tried, and ultimately failed.

This is a book about people needing each other. There is no shame in that; there is no more basic human condition, for without each other, we have nothing.

I began writing accounts of my interactions with people who had called 911 for help when I realized that my position exposed me to worlds that most of us would never experience. It is an honor to be allowed into a person's home, or into their lives when away from home, during a moment in time when their need is greatest, and is not something to be taken lightly. There is dignity to be found in just about every encounter we experience, and the people I have helped are the root of inspiration for this book. Their stories help unravel the mysteries of the human condition, and by telling them I hope to create a better understanding of the people we share this existence with, and how our differences need not keep us separate, or alone.

Some of the stories that follow are disturbing, others heartfelt, and many will leave you with a grin or scratching your head, much like I would do when responding to people's emergencies in the city of Providence, Rhode Island.

The people at the other end of the 911 calls are what matter. I am simply telling their stories.

Few are fortunate enough to be allowed into the innermost essence of others. Being one of the few has made my experiences more vibrant and my understanding of the people I share this time on earth with far deeper than I would have ever dreamed possible. Most of us get through our lives sharing ten percent or less of the thoughts that run through our minds. In times of crisis, that ten percent expands exponentially; the whole person is exposed. Sharing these experiences not only with the people who need help, but with my family, the people I respond with, and even the city itself, gives me the opportunity to be a better husband, father, friend, and firefighter.

Even now, somewhere somebody is in trouble, a call is being made, a dispatch transmitted, lights flashing, bells tipping, horns blaring . . .

CHAPTER 1
SEPTEMBER

Humanity (or Lack Thereof)

When she regained consciousness, he tightened the noose. Then he punched her in the face and waited for her to pass out. She did. A few minutes later he tightened the noose again. Eventually he grew bored and let her go, telling her she would never leave him. She called her mother, who called us, 911. I found her standing outside a three-decker in South Providence. Her two-year-old son cried hysterically in his grandmother's arms, screaming for his mother. I walked her toward the rescue; my partner met us with the stretcher. She lay on it, too dazed to speak, cry, or anything. She had been held captive for four hours and tortured. Outside her apartment life went on. The sun was bright, kids enjoyed the last few days of their summer vacation, construction workers worked on a stone wall a few houses down, oblivious to the horror a few feet away. I took her to the hospital. I hope she recovers.

Kellie

She looked sick, but then so many of them do after a long weekend. Providence College has its fair share of parties. Inside the health center the guys from Ladder 3 finished taking vital signs and gave me the preliminary report.

Nelson, who looks a lot like Wayne Newton, gave me the story.

"She's twenty-one, started throwing up last night at midnight. No medical history, doesn't take medications, and has no allergies. She seems a little confused."

Usually our college-age patients walk to the rescue, but not her. Her name was Kellie, her Irish name as beautiful as her face. She tried to answer my questions but her words were garbled. I became worried about her condition; we transported her immediately to Roger Williams Medical Center. Renato drove in his usual way, meaning I never felt a bump or turn in the road. En route, Kellie started to have seizure-like activity. As she vomited I handed her a basin. She didn't understand what it was and threw up on herself instead. She shook as I held the basin to her face, then fell back on the stretcher when I let her go. Her eyes couldn't focus on mine. I put her on a non-rebreather with high flow O_2 and let her rest. I felt her skin was cool and damp as I swept the hair from her eyes.

The nurse at the hospital took my report and immediately got her into a room, where she was seen by the doctor on call. I heard them mention a bleed as I washed the sweat and vomit from my hands. I had just taken off my gloves to do the report when she got sick. Five people were working on Kellie as I left. The doctor said it was probably a head bleed from an injury or meningitis. I hope it's meningitis and whatever got on me has been washed away.

Get Well, Kellie

The chief called at 2200 hours and told me to report to Roger Williams Medical Center. Kellie has bacterial meningitis and I was exposed. I had hoped she didn't have a bleed in her brain but I never expected this. Viral meningitis is bad, but not deadly. Bacterial meningitis kills.

It seems every year I read in the paper some poor kid who came to college and caught this bacteria somehow and died. Kellie's family is with her in the intensive care unit. She is intubated and fighting the infection but is in critical condition. I'll find out tomorrow if she lives or dies. As for me, I've taken a big dose of Cipro and should be all right. The medicine makes me sick, but not as bad as Kellie. I'm staying on duty until the morning.

Good News
It appears that Kellie may pull through. She has been extubated and woke up for a little while. She knew who she was and where she was but wasn't quite sure what had happened. She is lucky. Her roommates made her seek medical attention instead of going to sleep, which is what she wanted to do. The infection was caught before doing irreparable damage. Six firefighters and about forty staff and students were given antibiotics as a precaution. Her roommates saved her life. I love a happy ending and hope things continue to improve.

Tiny Package
What struck me first was the beauty of her children. A boy and two girls, anywhere from two to six years old, greeted me at the door. We exchanged shy grins and smiles as I made my way toward the patient. The guys from Engine 11 were already there and had assessed her vital signs and condition. She was weak and experiencing heavy vaginal bleeding. Her dark skin managed to look pale and translucent, and I could see her hair under her scarf was damp with sweat and matted to her head. The kids watched us fearlessly as we did our work. Jerry told me her vitals were stable, that she had a miscarriage. I wondered how he knew.

"The fetus is on the shelf," he said, deadly serious.

I looked toward the direction of his gaze at a tissue, neatly folded in half. Renato had the patient on her feet and with help from Jerry and the other guys was helping her out to the truck. I was alone for a moment with the kids and the fetus. The woman's husband walked in. He spoke English so I told him we were taking her to Women and Infants Hospital, a two-minute trip.

"I know," he said, not arrogant but demanding. "I'll follow in my car."

He left the fetus to me and walked outside. The kids were no longer smiling. I think they sensed my trepidation. A girl of about fourteen gathered them to her and they all left the room. I picked up the tissue and anxiously peeled back the top layer. Last night's Cipro made my stomach feel queasy, but this was overwhelming. I'd seen pictures of aborted fetuses, but this was altogether different.

I was mesmerized for a moment, surprised by the effect the fetus-shaped mass had on me. Somebody had washed it off and gently placed it on the tissue. I saw the eye; the head was separate from the body. I cradled the tissue in my hands and walked outside.

Expect the Unexpected
"Is that French?" I asked my patient.

"Oui," he replied.

"Did you learn that in Haiti?" I asked, making assumptions because of the color of his skin and prior experience.

"No, Montreal." His eyes rolled back in his head and he started shaking.

"He's seizing," I told Renato who had to pause his attempt to establish an IV. Slowly the tremors ceased and he opened his eyes. This time he spoke Russian.

"Is that Russian?" I asked with a smile.

"Of course, comrade!" he replied, then spoke Swedish, which I recognized from my grandmother who came directly from there two generations ago. "I know how to ask for toilet paper in ten languages," he laughed.

During transport I learned that he was a successful actor who did a lot of TV work in the seventies and some movie and stage stuff since. If you watch TV Land and catch a rerun of *Good Times* or *Laverne and Shirley* you will see him. I wondered why he landed in a methadone clinic. The answer was not what I expected. He has end-stage liver cancer and will die soon. His doctors suggested methadone as pain relief.

We had a nice conversation while traveling the five miles to Roger Williams Medical Center. I used to tread gently around dying people but have learned from them that they have no time or patience for bullshit. He told me if not for his Christian beliefs he would have already committed suicide. I understood. We shared our opinions of the afterlife and a special bond was formed. When we arrived at the hospital I said good-bye.

Some days I feel like the luckiest person alive.

9-11-06
I don't take for granted the things I have, my beautiful wife and kids, family and friends, good health and all that goes with it. I am more fortunate than most. That it could all end suddenly as it did for those poor souls five years ago is something I will never forget. Their lives ended that day, and a little of me went with them.

We are never truly safe; it could all be gone in an instant. I still have this instant, and in honor of those who perished I'll make it the best moment of time that I can.

Overdose

A guy my age, dressed only in boxer shorts, was lying on the bed in a puddle of vomit, a couple of syringes next to him. The person who called us stopped CPR when she saw us and walked out of the room. Renato got the bag-valve device, hooked it up to the portable oxygen tank I had carried to the fourth floor, and started bagging. I got the IV setup ready.

The tourniquet should have made his veins stand out but didn't. I fished around his left arm for a while, didn't find anything, and pulled the needle out. As soon as I did, blood leaked from the site. I guess I had a vein but didn't realize it. Narcan negates the effects of narcotics. I would rather administer it through an IV, but intramuscular or subcutaneous does the trick. I pinched the skin near his triceps, drove the needle home, and pushed the plunger. Two milligrams usually does it.

The guys from Ladder 4 and a Providence police officer joined us in the room. Renato kept bagging. A few minutes later the man started breathing on his own. He denied drug use but the evidence was overwhelming. I let him get dressed and walked him to the truck. On the way to the hospital he told me he was going away to rehab on Thursday to get some help. I told him he was seconds away from death. Thursday was almost too late.

Blood Money

She was getting ready to close for the night when a man wearing a hooded sweatshirt suddenly appeared at the drive-thru window. Instead of stepping back, the girl tried to stop him as he tried to pry the window open with a screwdriver. She failed. He forced the window open and went for the cash drawer. Again she tried to stop him. He grabbed a handful of her hair, pulled her head toward the window, and stabbed her in the face with the screwdriver. Luck was all that saved her left eye. She will be scarred for the rest of her life. She saved the company about eighty dollars with her heroics. The thug got away with the fives and ones. Tens and twenties littered the floor, covered with her blood.

There is true evil walking among us. I see it all too often.

Love Doctors

She didn't want to come out of the bathroom. I could hear her wheezing from behind the closed door. Her husband finally talked her out; we gave her an albuterol treatment to help her breathing. She had been crying. As the medicated mist began to work and her airway opened she began to relax. She forgot her inhaler at her friend's house, where they had spent the evening having a few drinks and some laughs.

I tried to get her to go to the hospital but she didn't want to go. They had a great night with their friends but as often happens with married folks on a Friday night, a stupid argument got out of hand and it looked like their night would end badly. During the argument she had an asthma attack. Her husband called 911 because he didn't know what else to do.

Me and Renato sat at their kitchen table as she finished the medication. We talked a while and had some laughs. By the time we left, the couple had ended their fight and couldn't wait to get rid of us so they could "get down to business." As we drove away I saw the lights go down in their tiny second-floor apartment.

Home

"Engine 11 to Rescue 1, bring some sheets and the stair chair." I keyed the mic and answered.

"Rescue 1 received, on scene."

The apartment house used to be a one-family place in what used to be a prestigious part of Providence. Peeling paint covered the ornate entryway that protected the carved oak doorway from the weather. We passed under the scrollwork, through the doorway toward our victim. Residents peered from the cracks of their partly opened and chained doors lining the hallway.

The guys from Engine 11 had opened the windows inside, forcing the putrid air down the stairs we were climbing. I pulled my T-shirt over my nose and mouth and entered apartment 6. Anna waited, lying in a pool of urine, her legs covered with feces.

"I fell off the toilet," she told me. I asked her how long she had been on the floor.

"Just a couple of days."

I checked for any bleeding or gross deformity before trying to move her. The clean white hospital sheet I placed over her was a sharp contrast to her under things, years old and yellowish grey, whatever color the material once held washed away. We managed to get her onto the stair chair, a long a laborious ordeal inside an environment we found reprehensible yet Anna called home. The guys carried her into the fresh air toward the rescue as I took note of her living conditions. Refrigerator empty. Closets empty. Floors and walls covered in filth, rat and mice droppings swept to the corners, displaced cockroaches scurrying for cover, no room to hide in walls already full.

Anna begged me not to take her away from her home. She told me she just needed to tidy up and get some rest. I felt like I betrayed her when I put in my report that she needed intervention, her living conditions unfit for humans.

Real Heroes

Every day the news comes home, "American soldiers killed in Iraq or Afganistan." Every day some poor soul's family confronts the fear they have kept hidden, their loved one is gone forever. Most of us watch from the sidelines as somebody's son, brother, wife, or husband boards the plane toward war. We watch from the safety of our living rooms the everyday heroes who fight this war for us. My brother is a member of the 1207th Transportation Company of the Rhode Island National Guard. It's his turn. His wife and four kids will wait until next September for him to come home from Iraq. There are some long days ahead. Be safe, brother.

Vacation
Vacation is almost over; I'm looking forward to getting back to work. This week went too fast. Providence managed to survive without me. Thursday will be here soon enough, we'll start over then.

Overwhelmed
We have six rescues in Providence, a city of 175,000. On the best days the pace is unbearable; days like today are truly impossible.

At 0852, Rescue 2 responded to the north end for an overdose. They found a naked man screaming next to the railroad tracks. He had been doing coke all night and decided to climb one of the high-tension electrical towers that power Amtrak's high-speed trains. In the dead of night, probably around three or four, he touched the wrong wire. He was knocked unconscious, his melted skin fused to the nylon warm-up suit he had been wearing. Nobody saw him until the morning. He was out of his mind when help arrived. The rescue crew had to wrestle him to the ground and restrain him. They were covered with his dead, smoldering skin for their troubles. They were being treated at the same hospital as their victim for exposure to whatever disease the man was carrying.

Rescue 5 went out at 0910 for an emotional woman who was acting violent toward her family. They managed to get the woman into the rescue. Moments later she vomited into the bucket Teresa had just handed her. Among other things she has hepatitis C. The vomit sprayed from the bottom of the pan into Teresa's eyes. She was treated at the same hospital as the woman, hard plastic lenses attached to her eyes while they flushed them with sterile saline from an IV bag. The process took three hours, leaving us with four rescues.

Another rescue went out for repairs for the morning, leaving us with three. The calls for help were nonstop. Rescues from surrounding towns called in to Providence to pick up the slack. Some people waited thirty minutes and more for help.

Tale of Two Cities
The call was for a seventeen-year-old pregnant girl with trouble moving. We were greeted at the door by the seventeen-year-old girl's two-year-old son. Another teen girl led us upstairs into a bedroom where our victim rested. She said her neck was stiff and she couldn't walk. I had her move her head from side to side, then up and down. She did it but said it hurt when she moved and had to go to the hospital for some muscle relaxers. I have given up arguing with people.

"Where are your shoes," I asked. She reluctantly walked down the stairs of her rent-subsidized apartment. During the two-block ride to Rhode Island hospital I copied her information from the state medical card she gave me. I noticed on the lower left edge of the card her co-pay arrangement: Emergency room co-pay, $0. Prescription co-pay, $0. Office visit co-pay, $0. Taxi ride to the emergency room by an advanced life-support rescue, dispatch of Engine 13 with four firefighters to assist with a potentially serious problem, $0.

I asked her why she didn't have friends or family take her to her doctor's office. She stared at me with a blank expression and ignored me. The state's Rite Care program provides full health care for children and their caregivers until the child turns eighteen.

Later that night we were sent to I-95 north at the Thurbers Avenue curve for a vehicle into the Jersey barrier. A car had lost control on the wet, slippery highway while navigating the tough curve in the road. The car was totaled, both air bags had deployed. Standing in front of the wreck was a twenty-year-old girl, covered in glass and holding the back of her head. We got her into the rescue. I automatically assumed we would take her to the emergency room, but she adamantly refused.

"Why?" I asked. "You might have a concussion."

"I don't have health insurance," she said. Rachel was driving home from work, traveling from New Haven to New Bedford after her shift. She was tired from working twelve hours and commuting two. Her employer didn't offer health care. She was out of school, living in an apartment with her friend, and barely making ends meet. The car was her roommate's. She should have been seen that night at the emergency room but knew the bill collectors would be relentless in their pursuit of payment. I had her sign a form stating she refused transport against medical advice, and then led her to a state police car. They got her off the highway to a safe place where she waited for a ride home.

CHAPTER 2
OCTOBER

Disaster

A car bomb exploded in Kennedy Plaza, killing eight and injuring almost two hundred, eighty critically. I left headquarters at 0844 and headed toward the disaster. En route a suspicious package was found, twenty feet from my planned entrance to the incident. I had to wait.

Walking wounded from a busload of tourists wandered the area looking for help as we staged a safe distance away. Some bled to death where they sat. Soon, the bomb squad cleared the area and we went in, establishing treatment area Bravo. A fifteen-year-old kid walked up to me and grabbed hold and wouldn't let go. He had a four-foot rod impaled through his shoulder. Dozens of firefighters were on the scene directing and transporting victims toward the four treatment areas. I extricated myself from the kid with the impaled rod and tried to get some supplies and help into my area, but radio communications were impossible.

I sent Renato into the thick of things to round up some backboards, bandages, IV setups, and manpower. While he was gone, ten more patients flooded into my area. I had nothing to give them, no help, no care, no time. I separated them into two groups, red for life-threatening injuries and yellow for those who could wait a few more minutes. The kid with the bar through his body ended up with the yellows. Other people looked worse.

Ten minutes passed. The wounded were restless and starting to panic. Kenny Prew, the officer of Ladder 3, miraculously appeared through the madness with a crew of four. He immediately saw my predicament and got to work. I was able to procure some ambulances from a staging area that the EMS commander had set up, just outside the red zone.

After about a half hour things started to get organized. My patients were reassessed and loaded into the ambulances to be sent to the transportation sector that sent them to the appropriate facility. In ninety minutes, 185 victims were triaged, treated, and transported away from the bombing scene. Seven of the eight dead were infants, their bloody bodies strewn about the area in pieces. A steady rain fell, creating a stream of blood that flowed through the area.

Four hundred people took part in the bomb simulation. It was the biggest drill in the history of Rhode Island. I learned a lot yesterday. I learned that I never want to be involved in a real bombing.

Trivial
He looked dead. Covered in dirt, unmoving, barely breathing. A passerby saw the crumpled heap while driving through the construction site and called 911. A massive highway improvement project is underway in Providence. Our victim collapsed there, a few feet off of Eddy Street, under a bridge. I checked for a pulse, found one, and helped Renato load him onto the stretcher. It was Kevin, a homeless alcoholic I know well.

We put him into the rescue and headed for Rhode Island Hospital, three blocks away. Kevin remained comatose en route, didn't even flinch while I started an IV. His vital signs were stable but he was completely unresponsive. I turned on the exhaust system in back but it was too late; the smell of stale piss, shit, and vomit had permeated my skin and clothes. I would be reminded of Kevin for hours.

Renato backed into the rescue bay. I got out and swung the rear doors open. As I pulled the stretcher out of the truck my patient sat straight up, looked me in the eye, and said, "WHO WAS THE GUY . . . THAT PLAYED THE CAPTAIN . . . ON *SEA HUNT*?" I dropped the wheels to the pavement and answered, "Lloyd Bridges!"

Kevin fell back onto the stretcher and we wheeled him in.

Chickens

"I didn't know that flies could live inside of a refrigerator," I said to my partner for the night, Ryan. He stood in the center of the room, careful to not rub against any walls. My patient, a fiftyish Cambodian woman, looked in the fridge again, then shut the door. Her family had gathered around her in her tiny upstairs bedroom. Blood streamed down the right side of her face, probably an injury from a fall. The woman opened the refrigerator again; a fly escaped, then she closed it and went over to a window and looked out, ignoring us.

"She's been drinking again," said a man, probably her son. I'd be drinking too if I had to live in these conditions. What to me is absolute squalor is to this woman paradise. People from her country have experienced horrors we can only imagine. I have taken this lady to the hospital before. I asked her about her country. She told me.

"I was lucky to make it to the refugee camp," she said as she recalled her childhood. "I hid in the woods when the soldiers came. I had eleven brothers and sisters. The soldiers killed them all, cut off their heads. They treated my family like chickens in a pen and cut them down. I watched from my hiding place as they killed my parents."

I think she was referring to the Pol Pot regime. She spent the next ten years of her life living in a tent with tens of thousands of other refugees, scrambling for food and medicine. Eventually she made it out and landed in Providence.

I cleaned the laceration with some peroxide, put a bandage over the wound, and made my way out of the house. I saw that the chickens that used to live in the kitchen cabinets were gone. The doors were back in place, the chicken wire thrown outside.

Day and Night

He sat on a wooden kitchen chair, incoherent, strings of drool and snot swinging from his nose and mouth as he swung his head from side to side. A few empties were at his feet, but I didn't think that was the problem.

"Is he diabetic?" I asked the people in the room. A woman of about fifty answered yes. The guys from Engine 3 got the stretcher from the rescue and brought it to the door. I wanted to get him into the truck to begin treatment. It wasn't easy.

"He don't need that. What you abusing him for?" asked one of the men in the room, agitated. He was a big guy, his distrust for the six middle-aged white guys who had invaded his place in the heart of the projects obvious. He glared at us as the other folks started to squirm. I wish I didn't notice that they were all black, but I felt the racial tension begin to rise. I have seen situations get out of control and racial divisions become an issue.

"If anybody has any suggestions I'm all ears," I said as the guys held the patient down and fastened the straps. "If this is a diabetic emergency, we can help him." The angry man relented, everybody relaxed, and we got the patient to the truck.

His glucose level was 10. I couldn't believe he wasn't unconscious. He fought hard, his brain screaming for nourishment. I drew up some glucagon, mixing the sterile water with the dry medication, then injecting it into his triceps muscle. The patient fought harder. Somehow Engine 3 held him still while Renato started an IV. I gave him 25 grams of dextrose through the IV and waited for it to work. He still struggled, but as his glucose level rose he returned to his normal self. The transformation was incredible. He didn't want to go to the hospital but I insisted. He gave in and we transported him to the emergency room. His friends watched silently from the doorway as we drove away.

Skin Deep

The wounds on his neck and wrist didn't look bad. I sat him on the bench seat next to the stretcher. The police asked him some questions. "Can you give me a description?" one of the cops asked.

"Three black guys."

"How much did they take?"

"About eighty dollars."

"Which way did they go?"

"I don't know."

One of the cops started speaking to my patient in Spanish. Indignant, the little Mexican guy on the bench sat up straight and said, "I speak English!" The cops left. On the way to the ER I asked what happened. All the courage Tony had mustered started to crack. His lower lip trembled, tears started to flow. He was ashamed. I didn't know what to do. Tony regained some of his composure and spoke in a shaky voice, barely under control.

"I was walking up my driveway." He talked while looking out the rear windows of the speeding rescue. "Fast! It happened so fast," he said. "One of them held me from behind and choked me. Another had a knife. He put it to my wrist and laughed, then sliced my skin open. Again and again!" I looked at the wounds on his wrist. They didn't seem superficial anymore. These cuts were deep.

Tony started to weep, covering his eyes with his shirtsleeve. The nice white shirt he wore, freshly pressed earlier in the evening, was ruined.

"Then he put the knife to my throat and wouldn't let go. They all laughed."

"'How does it feel to breathe your last breath?' one said and pressed the knife harder. I could feel the blood drip down my neck. I thought I was going to die!" Tony lost it completely then, cried uncontrollably until we pulled into the rescue bay. He was mumbling in Spanish now, the bravado he had shown earlier gone. I considered calling the police back, telling them that Tony had been robbed not only of his money, but his pride and dignity as well. If ever there was a hate crime, this was it.

I put Tony on a stretcher and backed out of the way as Rescue 3 rolled past with a level 1 trauma. Two guys were in critical condition after being stabbed in a barroom fight downtown. It occurred to me as I gave the report to Marie, the triage nurse, that this monstrous act would be reported as just another assault and robbery.

The other stabbing victim was rolling in as I was walking out. Tony sat on the stretcher staring into space, unaffected by the chaos surrounding him, but crippled from the turmoil within.

Déjà Vu

Hit and run. It is an epidemic in Providence. People come here from poor countries looking for work. They have no intention of staying here and starting a new life; rather they are here for the money, most of which is sent back home.

What little they keep for themselves is used for rent and food and if, there is enough left over, a car. Often, there is no money for insurance or registration, and a driver's license is impossible. It is easier to drive away and hide, or abandon a cheap vehicle that is on the road illegally, than face the consequences of their irresponsible actions.

John and Regina were minding their business driving on Academy Avenue when another car hit them, forcing them into a utility pole. I arrived on scene, noted the particulars of the accident, immobilized John on a long board with a cervical collar, and put him into the rescue. We moved him onto the bench seat and strapped him in. He said he was okay, but his neck hurt. His wife of fifty-three years, Regina, was next. We put her on the stretcher next to John and transported them to Miriam Hospital at their request.

For us it was an average run, something we do every day. For John and Regina it was a major incident. I found out later that John had broken his neck. He was in a brace for six weeks.

Five months later I was called to a beautiful home on Benefit Street. An elderly person had fallen, the radio said. Sitting on the couch was an eighty-two-year-old female holding her head, small streams of blood dripping between her fingers.

"What happened?" I asked. Her husband walked into the room. I looked at him, then her, then him again.

"She saved my life," the man said. "I was carrying the laundry down the stairs for her, I tripped and fell over the railing. If she didn't stop me I would have been killed!" The woman smiled at her husband and said her head hurt.

"It's not every day a two hundred and twenty pound man falls on you," she said. I looked at the stairway where the accident happened. I couldn't believe how lucky these two were. The man fell over a railing onto a landing, then tumbled down eight more steps, landing on his wife. When

I got them into the truck, the man on the bench seat on a backboard, the woman on the stretcher next to him, it hit me. "Haven't we done this before . . . ."

Where's the Remote?

"I am not going anywhere."

"You took ninety pills."

"Yeah, but I threw up."

"But you wanted to kill yourself."

"That was this morning, I'm okay now."

"I have to take you to the hospital."

"I'm not going."

"I'm not leaving without you."

"Well make yourself comfortable, there's a good movie on."

She was lying in her bed, in her pajamas. Her speech was slow and she looked glazed. Her mother called us when she found out her daughter had overdosed.

"I'm leaving; I don't want to see what they have to do," said the mother.

"What do we have to do?" I asked.

"What the last guys did. Tackle her, tie her up, and drag her to the hospital."

"I'm not tackling anyone," I said.

"She won't go willingly," said the mother.

I pulled up a seat next to the patient.

"Where's the remote?" I asked the girl. She chuckled, I chuckled, the mother stormed out. After five minutes of "negotiations," I walked her out to the rescue. She suffered from severe depression. Her medication didn't seem to be working. She was worried that she was going to miss her radiography class, her "A" average might suffer. I wish I could have spent more time with her; we hit it off pretty well. I told her about my daughters who were around her age.

"You are not alone, everybody has problems," I said. I think it helped. We walked into Rhode Island Hospital together. She will get a psychological evaluation and may have to spend a few weeks in a psychiatric hospital. They may pump her stomach. I hope not.

Sacrifices

The 1207th is firmly entrenched at Tallil Air Base, Iraq. My brother, Bob, called from there today to catch up on things. The constant hum of generators, rattle and crack of small arms fire and mortar rounds, and the roar of .50-caliber machine guns have replaced the sounds of home — my nieces and nephews playing (fighting), birds in the morning, crickets at night, and the precious quiet moments that we all take for granted.

The sacrifices our men and women in the armed forces are making cannot be understated. I hope that when their friends and families gather around the dinner table, the game, parties, or whatever it is that brings them together, instead of seeing an empty space, they see the person that should be there, and they hold their heads high and realize how fortunate they are to know them. I know I do.

Spanish Lesson

Today, Renato is teaching me how to say, "What's the matter with you?" in Spanish.

Homeless Alcoholics

To drink and die on the streets of Providence cannot be how so many envisioned their future. What dreams that once filled the heads of the homeless alcoholics who wander the city were replaced by cheap booze and the never-ending need for more years ago. A community of lost souls exists, their plight ignored by respectable citizens who pass them by each day without a second thought. Some panhandle, some steal, some collect government benefits. They all do whatever it takes to survive.

They know each other from chance meetings in homeless shelters, street corners, and emergency rooms. A wary friendship exists as long as the alcohol flows. Once the bottle is empty the quest begins again; friendship forged in desperation becomes secondary to survival. These are lonely lives lived by lost souls, an existence sane people cannot imagine.

Has society failed them, or have they failed society? It is a question I often ask as I transport one after another to the area emergency rooms. Time and time again the ritual is performed. Through the years I have come to know many. Cowboy, after years surviving on the streets, finally found dead in a Dumpster. Sivine, a Vietnamese refuge who dined in the trash cans that line Broad Street, dead in a field. Armand lost his frostbitten fingers one year, his toes another. He liked to sleep under the stars after a night of drinking. They found his body floating next to the pier near the hurricane barrier. Russell, a living corpse, survives on the streets by using Rhode Island Hospital as his personal hotel and the Providence Fire Department his taxi service. Curtis stayed sober for a year or so but has returned, drinking with a vengeance. Debra manages to put on her makeup at the shelter every morning; by afternoon she is drunk again, her tears leaving black trails down her cheeks, urine soaking her clothes. Chris has been missing for a while. I wonder if he is dead, sober, or waiting to make his triumphant return. John has been sober for years now. I see him from time to time. He is pleasant, a little reserved but sober. His drinking career ended the night he drank furniture polish looking for more when the booze ran dry. His friends let him do it and laughed when we took him away, comatose.

There are many, many more. Desperate people do desperate things. There is a lot of desperation lurking beneath the polished surface of the Renaissance City.

Why are these people allowed to roam the streets? Their behavior is habitual, suicidal, and reprehensible. Every day the emergency rooms treat the regulars. Russell alone has cost the hospitals and state and federal government millions of dollars during his drinking career. He takes from society and gives nothing in return. The combined cost caring for these individuals is astonishing. The homeless alcoholics drink until they can drink no more, then either they or a concerned citizen calls 911 for help and a rescue is sent. Nearby true medical emergencies occur, but the victims wait for help while a drunken person is given a ride to the hospital to sleep it off. Day after day, night after night they call.

There is no rehabilitation. There is no cure. There is no easy answer.

Who is responsible for this disgraceful situation? I am a guilty part of the machine allowing this debacle to continue. It is easier for me to put them in the rescue and dump them off at the hospital than to drive away and leave them to suffer the consequences of their actions. I have no intention of risking my livelihood if one of them were injured or died as a result of their self-inflicted condition.

The hospitals are also guilty. Day after day the patients are treated and released. The game is played over and over and has been for years. The Department of Health shares the blame. It is easier to maintain the status quo than develop a plan that will cure them or have them committed. The police department is also complicit. Why aren't the repeat offenders arrested for being drunk and disorderly or public drinking? Social services such as Crossroads try to help but simply cannot be held responsible for the actions of those who will not help themselves.

The fact that the drinking is funded largely by taxpayer money is another disgrace. Disability payments for alcoholic behavior fuel the very fires that caused the disability. Giving cash to people who have proven again and again that they are incapable of handling the responsibility is insanity.

Who has the courage to end the handouts and put these people where they belong: either prison or committed to a psychiatric facility? So far, nobody. Meanwhile, the bleeding of the health care system continues, and those unable to take care of themselves continue to die, drunk and abandoned.

I wrote this and submitted it to the *Providence Journal*. I made sure that six of the papers most popular columnists received a copy. Since then, Debra died; nobody claimed her body. Today, I found out that Russell is comatose at Rhode Island Hospital in critical condition. He had a seizure, fell, and smashed his head on the sidewalk he calls home. More lost souls have taken their place on the streets. I've never heard from any of the social commentators at the *Journal*, their stories apparently not worth the cost of the ink needed to print them.

Code 99

"Engine 11 to fire alarm. Code 99."

"Rescue 1, received, on scene."

Renato went to the rear compartment for the backboard. I opened the back doors and rolled the stretcher onto the street.

"Go," I told Renato. He disappeared through the chain-link gate and into the house. I got the blue bag full of medications and supplies and followed him in, leaving the stretcher thigh-high just outside the gate.

Inside, chaos.

An elderly woman lay on the floor next to a hospital bed, nightgown pushed over her waist. Not breathing, no pulse. A surprised look was frozen on her face. Family members, too numerous to count, ran in and out of the living room screaming. One guy walked into the middle of us, stepped over the dead woman, and went through some dresser drawers, looking for something. He found money, stuffed it into his pockets, and left the room. People kept screaming.

The guys had started CPR and were securing the victim to the backboard. I started to gather information.

"When was the last time anybody talked to her?"

"An hour ago."

"What medical condition does she have?"

"Arthritis."

"Where are her medications?"

Somebody handed me a basket full of pill bottles. I took them and headed for the truck. We got the lady inside, continued CPR, and ran the code.

"Renato, I need a line. Seth, you and Ollie keep on the CPR. I'm going to intubate."

Everybody had a job to do and we got on with it. I found the blue bag that held the ET kit, opened the zipper, grasped the handle and snapped the curved Mac blade in place. The bulb at the end went out. I got my ET kit assembled and tried to tube the patient. The bulb on the Mac blade, my favorite, went out as soon as I snapped it into place. I grabbed a Miller, longer and not as easy to use, for me anyway. I looked at Renato, who was on his third IV attempt. Nothing. I tried to intubate. In between the vocal vocal cords where the tube should entered the trachea never appeared, there was too much tissue and fluid blocking my view. The tube went down the wrong hole. I should never have tried it blind. I took the tube out after deflating the cuff and put an oral airway in her mouth. Seth continued compressions. Renato's forth IV attempt failed.

"I need a driver. Let's go," I said to Miles, the officer of Engine 11.

"I'll drive, but we'll have to leave the engine here," he said. I remembered that they were running with three instead of four. I didn't think leaving the engine unattended in this neighborhood was a great idea, but I would have left it right in the middle of the street if I thought it may have helped the patient.

"Just give me one of your guys," I replied. Seth left the back to drive the rescue, Miles drove the engine, Renato continued to attempt IV access, Ollie did compressions, and I handled the airway and bagging. We sped to Rhode Island Hospital. Somehow, I called the ER en route and told them what we had. They were waiting for us when we rolled in. We went directly to Trauma 2 where Megan, the resident, took my report.

"Eighty-year-old female last seen alive an hour ago found unresponsive by family. No CPR until EMS arrival at 2040. No IV access, no tube, asystolic, no blood pressure or pulse." Megan got to work without missing a beat. I listened while filling my paperwork. I didn't think the lady had a chance. After half an hour, they had a pulse and her blood pressure was 80/40. Not great, but something.

As we walked out of the ER Megan stopped us and said, "Great job, guys."

She meant it. Though we did our best, I thought our efforts were a total failure. Apparently, even though most of our efforts were futile, the CPR was enough to give the ER team a chance. I didn't think the lady would make it much longer, but at least her family would be able to sit with her when she dies.

Problems

Here's the story: Her daughter is under suicide watch and staying with her grandmother. Her husband, the suicidal daughter's stepfather, is in court being arraigned on possession of a loaded weapon (9mm). The stepfather is on probation from a previous conviction. The gun was in the truck the stepfather was driving (the mother's) because the suicidal daughter's mobster boyfriend gave it to the daughter because her father, a felon wanted in two states for rape charges, has been trying to contact his daughter who he molested. The husband was driving the mother's truck even though his left leg is useless due to an accident. The daughter had stashed the gun in the mother's truck. The stepfather was stopped by the police because he was driving erratically, possibly due to his useless left leg, and they found the gun. He was arrested. His wife came to district court to help her husband but was unable to see him. Her left eye started to ooze blood, the marshals called for a rescue, and I stepped in. We walked her out of the courthouse and into the rescue, where she told us her story. Me and Renato let her pour her heart out. She needed somebody to talk to. She said she has a tumor behind her eye that causes bleeding when her stress level rises. I hope she doesn't bleed to death.

Dignity

I didn't know how else to ask so I just said it.

"How much does she weigh?"

"Your stretcher won't break, they did it before," said her daughter. My stretcher is rated for five hundred pounds. My patient topped that, I'm sure.

"I don't want to hurt her if the stretcher collapses," I said. My patient remained motionless on the king-size bed, filling most of the mattress space. She was wheezing with rapid respirations. A crew of ten firefighters had assembled around the bed, a crowd had gathered outside, waiting to see the show. We had to get her to the hospital.

I stacked three hospital sheets, rolled them, and put them next to the patient. Her daughter climbed onto the bed and rolled her mom onto her side. The smell nearly knocked me over when the flesh was exposed, maybe for the first time in weeks. Her head and skeletal system moved to the side, most of her flesh stayed put. I helped stuff the gathered sheets under her until most of her girth was on top. We had to get her through the bedroom door into a hallway, through the outside doorway, down six cement steps, through a crowd, onto the stretcher, and into the rescue. Three firefighters got on each side of her, one at the head and one at the feet.

"On three," I said and we were moving. Once we got going it was hard to stop. At the bottom of the steps the stretcher waited. People gawked. The stretcher groaned but handled the weight.

"Nothing to see here!" said the daughter angrily to the crowd, who stood their ground as we worked. We got her into the truck and closed the doors. The crowd dispersed, the spectacle over for now. Renato and John stayed in back with me as we made our way to Rhode Island Hospital, steadying the stretcher because we couldn't lock it into place; it wouldn't fit. I called the hospital to get a large bed ready.

"I've got a sixty-year-old female, approx five hundred pounds, en route. We'll need a hospital bed, ETA three minutes," I said over the phone.

My patient turned her head and said, "I'm seventy-one," her pleasure that I thought she was ten years younger evident on her smiling face.

CHAPTER 3
NOVEMBER

Mabel

It took a while to spot her; she blended in with the litter covering most of the empty lot. I've learned to look closely when called to this address. With nowhere else to go, a lot of homeless people converge here. A couple of old chairs sat empty around a lonely tree. Used condoms, discarded clothing, broken glass, and Mabel were all that remained from the most recent gathering. It was cold, forty degrees or so, and getting dark. I walked up to the lump on the ground, bent over, and shook it. The lump stirred.

"Hey, buddy, let's go." I said. When I peeled back the blanket covering her face I realized it was a woman, one I had never seen before, not one of the regulars.

"What are you doing here?" I asked her.

"Sleeping."

"You can't stay here, it's cold and getting dark." She looked confused, then started to cry.

"What happened to me?" she asked.

"You're sleeping in an empty lot. You look intoxicated. I'm going to take you to the hospital," I told her.

"I just want to go home," she said.

"Where do you live?"

"Right off Prairie Avenue." She gave me the address and we walked her toward the rescue. Funny how quickly a desolate parking lot becomes inhabited when a spectacle appears, people wandered over, drawn to the scene by the flashing lights.

"Pull your coat together," I told her.

"I'm not cold."

"You pissed yourself and I don't want these people to laugh at you." She looked down and saw the wet spot between her legs. That was it. The tears ran like rivers down her dirty face as she closed her coat, covering the evidence. People stood to the side watching us with wary eyes as we stepped in and closed the door.

"I'm not like them," she said to me as we left the scene. She lived in a dreary three-story tenement house on one of the roughest streets in South Providence. I walked her past six or seven people who had gathered on the front steps and up the stairs to her second-floor apartment. When her sister opened the door I caught a glimpse inside. I saw why she found comfort with the homeless people she spent the afternoon with. Mabel walked in, gave me a shy smile as she closed the door, not wanting the gang partying in her front room to see the connection. I walked back outside, careful not to rub against the stairway walls.

Heart Attack

"Rescue 6 and Engine 7, respond to Memorial Boulevard for a male with chest pain."

We left the Atwells Avenue fire station at 2:04 p.m. John McGovern was driving, we were both working overtime. At 2:07 Engine 7 gave a report over the radio.

"Engine 7 to Rescue 6, fifty-two-year-old male, no history, with severe chest, diaphoretic at this time."

"Rescue 6, received."

2:11. We turned onto Memorial Boulevard. What should have been a bustling thoroughfare was a parking lot. In the distance a flurry of activity in front of the GTECH building caught my eye. Construction workers, truck drivers, and detail cops were directing the traffic frantically, clearing a path. Drivers of the cars and trucks blocking the route had no choice but to get out of the way. Fast. We flew through the path, inches between us and the stopped vehicles.

2:13. We stopped in front of the building. I saw the victim about seventy-five feet inside the garage, oxygen mask on his face, sitting, clutching his chest, two firefighters, Tim and Greg, helping him. Lieutenant Paul Picozzi met us at the rescue and helped with the stretcher. The guy was soaked with sweat and gasping for air. We had him on the stretcher and into the truck in two minutes.

2:15. We ran an EKG and attempted an IV. Greg gave him an aspirin, John got the man's blood pressure and heart rate. The truck was moving at 2:16. His EKG showed some ST elevation, indicating a probable inferior wall infarct. Another IV attempt failed en route. BP 158/100 with a pulse of 100. Greg slipped a nitro tab under the patient's tongue. "Let it melt, it should help."

2:20. We wheeled "Roger" into the ER. Donna was working triage. One look at the patient and she was on the Voicera announcing a medical team was needed in Trauma Room 3. I gave her my report as we rolled down trauma alley toward Trauma 3. Ashley and Leanne, two trauma RNs, waited.

2:22. Roger was on a trauma stretcher, Ashley and Leanne starting IVs while I helped Donna with another, more advanced EKG. Sara, the trauma doctor in charge, assessed the situation. She read the EKG when it was done, then ordered a heparin bolus, Plavix through the IV, a nitro drip, and a chest X-ray.

2:37. Seventeen minutes after arriving at the ER, thirty-three minutes after dispatch, Roger was in the cath lab with four IVs running and the proper meds on board.

Roger was lucky. His heart muscle began dying the minute his chest pain began. The construction workers and truck drivers who cleared the way, the cops who kept the road clear, the nurses, doctors, and firefighters worked perfectly together. A heart attack is basically the death of the heart muscle. Medical people have a saying: "Time is muscle." Roger will probably make a full recovery. I hope everybody involved in Roger's care understands how vital their role was.

As we drove away from the ER toward another run, both John and I agreed. This is the best job in the world.

Enough

4:12 a.m. It's late. Or early, depending on how you see things. Right now I'm seeing things as pretty dreary. I was at RI Hospital delivering my ninth intoxicated male of the night to the ER when a life flight landed on the helipad. A female, around sixty, was in critical condition, her husband, also critical being transported by land arriving soon. The trauma team worked on the woman as I left to pick up a twenty-two-year-old who vomited. The girl was a real bitch, wouldn't look at me, and barely answered my questions.

When I got back to the ER the woman was dead. Her husband in the next room will survive but will probably be paralyzed. They were out celebrating his birthday. Something happened, the car rolled, they were ejected. The usually hardened people who work in the ER were stunned. They went on, caring for the endless flood of patients marching through their door. The unfairness and cruelty of life amazes me.

I've been here for thirty-four hours and have four to go. No sleep, thirty-two runs so far. I can't wait for this to end, go home and kiss my wife, then fall asleep and hope the depression I feel is gone when I wake.

Out with the Devil

There was a pedestrian struck on the corner of Cranston and Bridgham. We were at RI Hospital finishing up at the triage desk. I keyed the mic.

"Rescue 1 to fire alarm, in service from Rhode Island, we'll handle Cranston Street."

"Roger, 1, you've got it."

Renato hit the lights and sirens and sped out of the ambulance bay. We both knew a lot of kids hung around that corner. A minute into our response Engine 3 gave their report over the radio.

"Engine 3 to fire alarm, advise Rescue 1 we have a seventeen-year-old male, conscious and alert with minor injuries."

"Rescue 1, received."

Renato slowed to a reasonable speed as we approached the scene. A young Hispanic guy sat on a curb holding his knee, squeezing it, trying to get more blood from the tiny scrape. A crowd had gathered, surrounding us. I asked the guy if he was hurt. Three people from the crowd answered for him.

"He needs a doctor!"

"Take him to the hospital!"

"What are you waiting for?!"

I looked at the knee and asked him what happened.

"I was riding my bike and the car ran into me."

"Did you run into the car or did the car run into you?"

The guy who was driving the car stood off to the side with the police. There was no damage to the bike or the car and only the slightest damage to the knee. The crowd continued their banter. Renato talked to them in Spanish; that quieted things for a while. Again I asked the patient, "Are you hurt?" Again the crowd started.

"He's hurt!"

"Get him to the hospital!"

"Hurry up!"

I had to walk away. I was talking to myself, something about lawyers, Jerry Springer, Democrats, Republicans, and morons, when Joe, the officer of Engine 3, pulled me to the side. He shook his head, took a deep breath, and said, "Repeat after me: in with Jesus," he exhaled sharply and said, "out with the devil," then walked back to the crowd. I'm not a religious man and I don't know about Joe, but he brought me back to where I needed to be. I walked through the crowd, back to the patient.

Good-Bye

This time she was dead. Facedown on her dirty mattress, hands purple. Her family stood outside the cramped bedroom door and peered in from time to time. I crawled onto the mattress and lifted her arm to feel for a pulse. Rigor mortis had begun. Her skin was like ice. No pulse. I backed off the mattress and stood in the tiny room, surrounded by tiny people, kids and adults. The flies that buzzed around the little refrigerator seemed bigger, slower, as though their time on earth was short. For the lady on the mattress, time had run out. What a miserable life, I thought, recalling her story of escape from the horrors of postwar Cambodia and the years of hardship in the refugee camps. Her escape into a pool of alcohol hastened her demise, which I imagine came as a relief for her.

"She's gone. I'm sorry for your loss," I recited to the people in the room. The littlest ones cried freely now, their fears confirmed by the giant in their grandmother's room. Only the kids spoke English. They interpreted for the adults, who shook their heads, no tears, just grim acceptance. The ability to feel had not been stolen from the younger generation by a repressive, brutal regime. Maybe their tears will help cleanse the memories their elders must endure. I left their home, probably for the last time, my services no longer necessary.

Russell

I knew he wouldn't make it much longer. I can't believe he lived for as long as he did. I can't say I'll miss him, or that I'm sad now that he's gone. I am a little concerned that I don't feel anything at all. I sometimes wonder if this job takes more than it gives.

Married Bliss

She could barely stand; he wasn't much better. They were down on the sidewalk at 390 Douglas Avenue. Somebody called us from their cell phone. A small cut over her right eye had stopped bleeding but the dried blood remained on her face.

The guys from Engine 12 helped them into the rescue. She started complaining immediately; he nodded out. This was my first call in eight days. Vacation is nice but ends too quickly.

"Wake up!"

He jumped and opened his eyes. "What happened?" I asked.

She answered. "Nothing happened. We don't have to go with you so let us out."

"You'll fall if I let you out."

"No I won't. If I do my husband will pick me up."

I looked at her "husband," out cold on the bench seat.

"Wake up!" They had all the signs of heroin addicts. She had just gotten out of detox at Roger Williams Medical

Center. He picked her up. From the looks of things, detox lasted until she reached the first package store or dealer. "How many bags?" I asked him, his pinpoint pupils giving up his secret.

"I didn't do heroin, I'm on eighty of methadone. I could do ten bags and it would feel like an aspirin," he said with pride.

"I could do twenty, no problem," she chimed in. They told me they just wanted to go home. Their address was a few blocks away. Rhode Island Hospital was packed, Miriam diverting, and Roger Williams a nuthouse.

"If I take you home, stay home," I insisted. They relaxed and held hands during the ride. He told me he had to catch a bus at six the next morning. "Where are you going?" I asked.

"Work."

Instead of bringing them to the hospital for babysitting, I took them home and watched them as they stumbled in.

Walking

She walked out of her house holding her belly. She was pretty, but looked tired. I was surprised to see her walking. I've noticed a lot of people who call 911 in the middle of the afternoon because of abdominal pain are either drug seekers, hypochondriacs, or worse.

This woman was different. I would have carried her even if she insisted on walking. We helped her into the truck and got her on the stretcher. She spoke limited English so I let Renato do the talking. The color drained from his face as he translated.

"She says her stomach started swelling last night at around three. The pain has been getting worse. She had chemo four weeks ago but the cancer spread to her liver. It started in her ovaries but keeps spreading. It's stage four now. She's in a lot of pain." I wrote the information onto the state run report.

The fact that struck me most was her age. Thirty-seven. She lay on the stretcher, closed her eyes, and rested during transport. A few tears were shed along the way. I don't know if they were tears of pain or hopelessness.

CHAPTER 4
DECEMBER

Party's Over

The party was in full swing for most of Thayer Street, but not so for Marissa. She sat on a curb in front of Starbucks, the shoes that once matched her party dress now splashed with mud and vomit.

"I just want to go home, take me home" she said to the guys from Engine 9. Whether or not she was aware that we were there to help her is unclear. I imagine all she could see was a blur. Fortunately for her, we showed up to take her "home" rather than somebody whose intentions were not so noble.

She was defenseless.

We carried her onto the stretcher, gave her a bucket and a towel, and drove toward Rhode Island Hospital where she would join twenty or so other intoxicated college kids. As I searched her small black bag for some ID I found a fancy silver flask, empty now, but carefully filled earlier with the cause of all her troubles. The ID lay under the flask—the picture on it showing a beautiful California student was a sharp contrast to the drunken wreck thrashing on the stretcher.

"I'm sorry, I'm sorry," she said over and over. I covered her with a hospital blanket but she kept pushing it away, unaware that her dress which cleverly covered her when sober now left nothing to the imagination. I wrapped her up as best as I could before wheeling her into an ER filled with cops, firefighters, patients, and hospital staff.

Addicted

She was eight months pregnant and sick, her skin pale and sweaty in spite of the cold night air. She tried to vomit but there was nothing left.

Just because you are pregnant doesn't mean you are no longer an addict.

A day ago she left the safety of Women and Infants Hospital, against their advice. She said she was bored. I say she went looking for heroin. The fact that we found her wandering the streets of South Providence at five in the morning did little to support her story.

"I need my methadone," she sobbed while shaking with convulsions. "Why won't anybody help me?" she cried as the tremors subsided. She dry heaved.

"Get in the truck," I said, helping her up the steps and into the rescue.

Some Days . . .

A drunken driver crashed into a minivan, damaging both vehicles. Nobody was hurt. The police officer on scene tried valiantly to have an officer who was equipped and trained to run a sobriety test respond to the scene but failed.

Friday night. Nobody working was qualified to administer the test. A city of 170,000 residents and countless thousands more visiting the colleges and clubs and nobody could administer a sobriety test. What to do? Call a rescue.

We picked the guy up a half mile away from Roger Williams Medical Center. He was in his early fifties and had attended his Christmas party earlier in the evening and somehow got lost in the capital city. Renato helped him to the rescue while I checked his car for damage. No windshield stars, no air bag deployment, no damage to the steering wheel. As I turned away from the car I saw a wallet on the ground next to the driver's door. There were plenty of twenties but no ID. The patient was sitting on the bench seat when I entered the truck.

"This is your lucky day," I said to him, handing the wallet over.

"What did you take my wallet for?" he demanded, slurring his words.

"I didn't, it was on the ground."

"No it wasn't. You took it out of my pocket," he said, angry now. I ignored him.

"What is your name?" He ignored me. "You have got to be the stupidest man on earth," I said. "You crashed your car and nobody got hurt, you got out of a DUI and had a wallet full of money returned to you, and still you act like an asshole."

"You're the asshole."

"Am not."

"Are too."

"Am not."

We arrived at the ER just in time.

Quiet
Anybody who works in the ER knows not to mention or even notice if things are quiet. When the torrent of patients that flow through the doors ebbs, disaster can't be far behind.

Saturday morning. Beautiful late fall weather outside, more staff than patients inside the sliding glass doors. Ten empty stretchers waited in the triage area, more lined the hallway of trauma alley. I had just dropped off an intoxicated patient and sat behind the triage desk for a while with Joanne, a lovely RN from England. We reminisced about last

Christmas Eve, a bloody mess we recalled, more heartache and suffering than joy visited upon the ER. I asked her how her plan to give goats to needy African families as Christmas gifts in lieu of presents was working. Before she could answer my portable crackled to life.

"Rescue 1, respond to the Rhode Island Hospital helipad for an incoming MedFlight."

"Rescue 1, message received."

"Duty calls," I said and walked out the doors and into the brilliant sunshine. The MedFlight ended up being cancelled, the victims of a head-on collision being transported by rescue. We went back in service and drove toward the station, hoping things remained the same, not that we noticed things were quiet, of course.

Two hours later, we returned to a different ER. Most of the stretchers were full, everybody was busy. The head-on collision had taken the life of two elderly ladies; the driver of the other vehicle remained in critical condition. It is amazing how quickly things change. Joanne, busy now, managed to take a minute to talk.

"Terrible thing," she said. "Two nice ladies, all dressed up. Their hair was done, makeup perfect. They must have been shopping." She shook her head and walked away. I walked my drunken patient through the madness toward the clinical decision unit, where he would be monitored until he sobered up, then released into police custody. He remained oblivious to the suffering surrounding us. Perhaps he knows something we don't.

Bad Trip
She sat on the love seat in a luxury suite at the Biltmore Hotel, swaying from side to side then front to back. She didn't struggle, but offered no help either. The cops there told me they found a suicide note on her laptop, an instant

message sent to the person she meant to meet in Providence. I think there was to be some sort of rendezvous. The person on the other end of the e-mail messaging contacted us when it became clear things were not going well. The address on the empty prescription bottle read Washington State, far from home.

The ninety Oxycontin that had been prescribed two days ago were gone. So were the thirty Oxycontin prescribed yesterday. Two empty bottles of fine wine sat next to an empty liter of top-shelf vodka. She was nearly unconscious as we wheeled her to the elevator to the lobby. Renato started a line once we were in the rescue, the guys from Ladder 1 hooked her up to the oxygen and got her vitals.

"80/40 with a pulse of 45," John Fallon said.

"I've got a line," Renato told me. Her glucose level was low, 44. As I got an amp of D-50 ready, Al Scott suggested Narcan.

"Thanks, Al," I said, handing the vial of D-50 to Renato and drawing up 2 mg of Narcan and 100 ml of thiamine. Once all the drugs were on board, we reassessed her condition. 90/60, pulse 68, glucose 136.

Better. The lethal dose of narcotics and alcohol was held at bay for now, but our patient was still critical. We transported her to Rhode Island Hospital, where she spent the rest of the night in a trauma room being constantly monitored. Her respirations and blood pressure remained unstable but she is expected to survive her ordeal.

A visit that held so much promise nearly ended with disaster. I hope she gets the help she needs and is able to start over.

What Her Father Carries
From *TIME* magazine, Letters to the Editor, December 11:

Re., "THE THINGS THEY CARRY" (Nov. 20,) on the tokens from home that the Marines from Kilo Company take into battle in Iraq: Since my dad is in the Army National Guard, serving in Iraq, I thought he would appreciate my telling you what he carries. It's a small Celtic cross. He got one for himself, my mom, me, my two brothers and my sister. We all wear them on chains around our necks – except he wears his with his dog tags. We wear them so we can keep him in our hearts, and he can keep us in his.
Catherine Morse
Hope, RI

Catherine is eleven. She made ornaments for her dad's Christmas tree that her mom boxed the day after Thanksgiving. The lights on the tree are battery operated. They will fade as the days toward Christmas march onward. I can't shake the image of a soldier in the desert looking at his Christmas tree and thinking of home, his hope dimming along with the lights.

Hang in, Brother. Your wife and kids are making all of us proud.

Cause No Harm
The car was demolished. The air bags had deployed and a wooden utility pole was lying on the ground, snapped off at the base. The people in the car had to be seen at the ER. Two boys claimed they weren't hurt; their mom was hysterical, claiming she had pain "everywhere." Pat, the officer of Engine 10, called for additional rescues. The mom went nuts, begging me to not separate her from her boys. The six-year-old was crying, his eight-year-old brother about to start.

"I have to take you to different hospitals," I explained to the boys' mom. "A pediatrician needs to check your kids for injuries." The boys had no signs of physical trauma but were emotionally traumatized. I asked each of them if they felt any pain at all, anywhere. They said no. The mechanism of injury suggested following state protocol: boards and collars for everybody, three separate rescues for transport. If the boys had hidden injuries and were not properly restrained during transport, my EMT license and livelihood could be in jeopardy. Lawyers can be an unscrupulous bunch.

The mother leaned off of her backboard and clung desperately to her kids, begging me not to separate them. The kids were sobbing and afraid. The mom's injuries appeared minor; the boys were more upset than anything.

Six of one, half dozen of the other, or something like that. I weighed my options, then decided to do the right thing.

Sometimes That Happens

"I don't know how he did it, but he knocked the refrigerator over," said the intoxicated man. "I think he hurt himself."

The third-floor apartment was decorated for the holidays. Two stockings were hung by the living room window, a small ceramic tree sat on an end table.

"Sometimes that happens," I said as I walked into the kitchen. The fridge was facedown on the floor. Another man was in a bedroom next to the kitchen, in bed, smoking. "What happened?" I asked.

"The refrigerator fell," he said.

"Sometimes that happens," I answered. "Are you hurt?" He looked at me with glazed eyes and kept on smoking. "Are you hurt?" I asked again.

"I'll be fine." With help from the guys from Engine 14, we stood the fridge back up. A call came in for a five-year-old with difficulty breathing a few streets away. We left, assuming that the guys would take care of themselves.

Changes
She apologized for calling us.

"I didn't want to bother you, but I can't stand the pain any longer." Her home was meticulous, nestled on a quiet street in the Mount Pleasant section of the city, surrounded by beautiful yet modest homes that showed the pride of their owners. The city has a few neighborhoods like this, though they are becoming scarce. She handled her pain well, as a lot of people from her generation are prone to do. No theatrics, just a matter-of-fact explanation of her problem. She insisted on walking to the rescue, turning out the lights and locking the door behind us.

She was born in 1920. I remarked that she must have seen a lot of changes. I don't know if she was looking out the back windows as we left her sanctuary and traveled through a more desolate part of the city toward Rhode Island Hospital. There isn't much activity at four in the morning; the old houses look much the same in the dim moonlight as they did in prior decades. When the sun rises and the city wakes, the real changes become clear. A few of the houses were still illuminated with Christmas lights.

"I don't think you will have to stay in the hospital for Christmas," I said, assuming her ailment could be treated without an extended stay.

"It doesn't matter," she said, sadness filling her voice.

"Why?"

"My husband passed away last year and I'm just waiting to join him. We were married sixty-four years; it's hard to live without him."

"You must miss him," I said.

"Terribly." As we neared the hospital, she told me of the greatest gift he ever gave her.

"As he neared the end he told me this: 'If I could live my life over again, I wouldn't change a thing.' That kind of love is what keeps me going. We had a wonderful life together." The truck stopped at the ambulance bay.

"He must have been a great man," I said.

"He was. He was a captain on the Providence Fire Department, Ladder 5 at Point Street."

Ghost of Christmas (Russell)

I still see him sometimes, standing at the pay phone at 1035 Broad Street, a slumped figure waiting for a ride to the hospital. Every day, sometimes twice he would call, claiming he had chest pains, a seizure, or was bleeding. Sometimes he told the truth and said he was drunk. Whatever the reason, we took him to the emergency room to dry out. The people there treated him well, gave him clothes when needed, cleaned him up if necessary and gave him his seizure medication. In his mind we were his family. His real family gave up on him years ago; we couldn't. Whenever he called we took care of him.

I don't blame him for abusing the system so blatantly. He was a survivor who used any means available to get by. We offered sanctuary; he took it. He became part of our routine, annoying but harmless. At times he was amusing. He knew he was dying and chose to let life go without a struggle. I wish he hadn't given up.

Rest in peace, Russell, and happy birthday. I hope you found what you were looking for.

Far but Close

Home. It's not a place.
It is the people we carry in our hearts.
Home can be found any place,
at any time.
Some people spend their entire lives
looking for home
and never find it.
Others know it,
feel it every day
and are not afraid to fight
and die for it.
Time spent away
from friends and family
strengthen bonds
that have already been formed.
The sights are not as clear,
the tastes and smells of home
become more difficult to recall,
but the love and respect
for those missing
only grows stronger.

Merry Christmas to all, especially my brother, Bob, and Hector from Rescue 2, PFD, who are serving our country in Iraq.

Scrooge

Peter said it best the day after Christmas. "I feel like a spaceship picked me up at my house and dropped me off on another planet." We were driving back to the station after dropping a girl off at the ER who called us because she didn't want to wait at Roger Williams Medical Center. The waiting room was full, so she decided that if she went home and called 911 she would get in faster at Rhode Island Hospital. I asked her for ID. She gave me the state Rite Care card.

I don't think I have ever seen a rescue on my street at home. The streets of Providence are different. We are glorified busses. The Red and White Taxi company. Three hundred bucks a trip at taxpayer expense. The abuse is unbelievable. I read in the paper today how advocates for the poor descended on the statehouse demanding more funding. That article was just below another story about obesity being a problem for poor families. That article was next to one about the guy who was shot to death Christmas Day in Providence. He was at a nightclub drinking and dancing at one thirty when somebody opened fire. Wrong place, wrong time. Now his two kids don't have a father. Christmas Eve, when I was home putting presents under the tree for Christmas morning, he was drinking and dancing at a nightclub with a long history of violence. It sounds like they didn't have a father to begin with.

CHAPTER 5
JANUARY

Code Red

"Engine 11 to fire alarm, we have a smoke condition." Miles could have been ordering a pizza from the sound of his voice, but everybody responding to Calla Street knew better. This was a working occupied house fire. Engine 11 arrived on scene and confirmed it.

"Code Red!" All companies responding to the fire had a job to do. The second arriving engine was responsible for the water supply. The first due ladder company needed to "get the roof." The third engine backed up Engine 11 and the second ladder started a primary search. Special Hazards did whatever the situation dictated and Division 1, the chief, was the incident commander. Rescue 1 arrived and established the EMS sector and waited for victims. Thankfully everybody got out of the house.

Seven or eight family members huddled together outside and watched their home burn. Renato got some blankets and handed them to the shivering people, a small comfort but one I'm sure was greatly appreciated. The fire started in a rear first-floor stairway and had reached the third floor by the time somebody noticed smoke and called 911. It spread fast and ended up in the loft. We had the stubborn blaze under control in about thirty minutes. Salvage covers were brought in to cover the family's valuables from further damage. When the smoke cleared they were allowed back into their home to collect some things, then the American Red Cross provided them with emergency lodging and food. There are hundreds of similar incidents every year in Providence.

Not Easy
It looked like he was walking under water. His frustration was obvious, the cause was not. They walked together toward the rescue, an attractive couple in their late twenties. She moved gracefully, taking her fluid movements for granted, as most of us do. He fought for every step he took.

"What's wrong?" I asked when he finally made it to the truck and sat on the bench seat.

"I can't move very well and my head feels heavy," he responded in a deadpan voice.

"Do you have any pain, especially near the eyes?"

"My left eye hurts and my vision is a little blurry," he answered me.

"How long have you felt like this?"

"This time, about two days. I'm worried it's getting worse."

"Do you take any medications?"

"Not now, but I was taking Copaxone until it made me sick."

"Were the daily injections the problem or the medication itself?"

"I think it was the medication," he answered, interested in my questions now.

"Have you tried Avonex or any of the other medications?" I asked.

"I don't like the side effects."

"When were you diagnosed?" I asked.

"Two years ago. You are the first person other than my doctor who knows what I'm talking about," he told me.

We talked during the trip to the hospital about his disease, multiple sclerosis. His frustration had more to do with being misunderstood than his symptoms.

"My wife's family thinks I'm lazy. My friends think I should work out more. I think I'm going crazy," he told me. He was in the process of being hired as a Providence police officer when his symptoms began. First he felt strange tingling sensations. Then pain in his eye and blurry vision. Next was the fatigue.

That was the worst part, he said. "I can't do a thing without being exhausted. I feel like a burden to my wife. Thank God for her, she has been great."

I did my best to give him something to be optimistic about but found it difficult to do. MS is a dreadful disease. His wife met us in the ER. I wished them well before going back to the truck; let them know that though it is a struggle, living with MS can bring them closer together. They appeared to have what it takes to survive the long, hard years ahead of them. As we drove away from the ER, I called Cheryl, my wife, and asked how she was feeling.

Serenity
I had lunch on Thayer Street, whole-wheat crust pizza with fresh mozzarella and plum tomatoes, and a ginger ale. The peaceful sound of a saxophone drifted through the rescue's windows. Sixty degrees on January 5. For almost twenty minutes we relaxed until an intoxicated male at a pay phone needed medical assistance.

Thirty Minutes
The usual suspects were in the empty lot at 1035 Broad Street, pointing toward the corner where Junior sat. He was slumped on the curb, obviously intoxicated. We had been dispatched to this corner for an intoxicated male. Thirty

seconds before we arrived on scene, somebody else called from a few blocks up with chest pain. Rescue 2 was coming from Hartford Avenue, six or seven minutes away.

"Let's see what's up the street," I said to Renato. We rolled past Junior to check on the chest pain. Inside a storefront was a guy about my age clutching his chest. I keyed the mic.

"Rescue 1 to fire alarm, we're diverting to 1089 Broad for the chest pain. Have Rescue 2 continue to 1035 Broad for the intoxicated male."

"Roger, Rescue 1. Rescue 2 receive?"

"2 received."

We helped the guy clutching his chest into the rescue. Steve, from Engine 10, started an IV while Renato ran an EKG. I got the guy's information from his brother, who stood in the doorway of the rescue as we worked. Forty-five years old, no medical history, doesn't take any meds, has no allergies, no illegal drug use or alcohol. He was sitting down writing something when the chest pain began. 158/94, pulse 86, pain scale 10/10, radiating up the left arm toward the jaw.

"I've got a line," said Steve. I gave the patient 325 milligrams of baby aspirin to chew, then a nitro tab to slip under his tongue. The initial four lead EKG showed some ST elevation. I waited for the results of the twelve lead. Renato read it out loud.

"Anterior wall myocardial infarct. You guys ready?"

He gave me the printout, then left the back to drive to Rhode Island Hospital. I called the triage desk en route. Leigh was waiting when we got there.

"Trauma Room 3," she said and led the way down the busy corridor. Dr. MacGreggor was in the room waiting along with Maggie. I told the doctor the story while Leigh and Maggie started another line and pushed the meds that the doctor ordered. Rob ran another EKG, which was identical to our findings. Thirty minutes from the time the patient felt the beginning of his heart attack he was in the cath lab. Everybody involved played a major role in saving the patients life. Even Junior, who got us going.

Madness

She sat on the stretcher in the back of the rig, a beautiful one-year-old with an air of royalty about her. She looked like the Queen of Sheba as she captivated her subjects: myself, her grandmother, and Danielle, my partner for the night.

It was the baby's birthday. During the party, she managed to get into a roll of toilet paper. When she grew tired of playing with it, she ate it. The grandmother saw that she was choking, tried in vain to clear the airway but couldn't. Somebody called 911. I had just arrived at the ambulance bay at Rhode Island Hospital when I heard the call.

"Engine 12, respond to 919 Douglas Avenue for an infant with an obstructed airway."

They didn't send a Providence rescue because we were all busy on other runs, as is often the case. Mutual aid companies respond to Providence thousands of times every year due to a dangerous shortage of rescues in the capital city. Six rescues handle calls from a city with an official population of 175,000 but is much more populous than that. Fortunately, I was able to clear the hospital quickly.

"Rescue 1 to fire alarm, clearing Rhode Island, we can handle Douglas."

"Roger, Rescue 1 at 1835."

Captain Morrocco gave Engine 12's report three minutes later.

"Engine 12 to fire alarm, advise rescue a one-year-old infant, airway was clogged but now is clear, respond Code C."

Just what I wanted to hear. We slowed to a reasonable speed and arrived on scene. I had released Engine 12 and was in back doing vitals on the queen when the side door opened suddenly and a man entered, screaming at the grandmother. He was out of control, slamming his fists on the roof while continuing his tirade. I stood from my seat and literally pushed him out the door. He continued his verbal assault on anybody who would listen, eventually venting his anger on the baby's uncle who was standing near the rescue.

"Rescue 1 to fire alarm, have the police and Engine 12 respond here."

"Do you have a nature?"

"Assault in progress outside the rescue."

I put the mic down and watched the man punching the side of the house we were parked in front of. He then ripped a drainpipe from the side of the house and began to walk back toward the rescue. I heard Engine 12's siren in the distance and could only hope they got to the scene before things got out of control. They did. The guy with the drainpipe stayed where he was as the four firefighters got out of their truck and came toward the rescue. I unlocked the door when Captain Morrocco knocked and told him what was going on. By that time, three police cruisers had arrived and had the guy with the drainpipe in custody.

It turns out that he was the little girl's father. Somebody had him on his cell phone and was telling him that his daughter was choking to death. He was fired up when he got to the scene. Ten minutes later everything was back to normal. The father wasn't arrested, the baby wasn't choking, the engine was back at the station, and I was doing my report. It was difficult to articulate what I believed to be an unsafe situation for the one-year-old girl without knowing all of the circumstances. If I have to come back to this address, I hope it's not because the baby is injured.

Some of us are held responsible for our actions.

Delivery

The Baby Jesus was coming but there was a delay. The mom had a diabetic emergency on the day she was to deliver. Her blood sugar level dropped to 26. Her family tried to get her to drink some orange juice with sugar but it only dribbled down her chin.

Engine 12 was first on scene. Lieutenant McCoart gave me his report when we arrived.

"Thirty-six years old, full-term maternity, diabetic with low glucose. Her family found her in bed unresponsive and soaked with sweat."

Renato got the stair chair from the back and I took the blue bag. The patient lay in bed, semiconscious in a bedroom at the top of the second-floor stairs. Three generations of caregivers surrounded her—her sister, her mother, and one of her daughters who was around ten.

"She managed to drink a little juice but she is still out of it," said her sister. Renato got a box of glucagon from the blue bag. Two vials were inside. He opened one containing 1 mg of solution, extracted it with a 3 ml syringe and a 22-gauge needle, then injected that into the other vial which contained the dry medication. He mixed the solution, sterilized an area on the patient's upper arm, and injected the medicine into her triceps muscle.

"Does she take any medications?" I asked the sister.

"Insulin, morning and night. She is also taking prenatal vitamins."

"Are there any complications with the pregnancy?"

"They are inducing labor today. She is having a boy, the first one in the family!"

I looked at all of the women in the room and thought how lucky the newborn baby was going to be. Spoiled rotten, I'm sure, but surrounded by adoring sisters, aunts, and grandmothers.

Our patient began regaining consciousness. She looked surprised when her eyes focused and she saw a room full of family and firefighters. After a few minutes we loaded her into the truck and transported her to Women and Infants, where she will stay until the delivery. I'm sure the family will be ready when the mother and son return.

Fathers
"You don't look depressed," I said to her as I walked past her and followed her counselor into the kitchen of the group home. She gave a hairy eyeball, directed at the counselor I'm sure, then walked to the rescue with Andrea, my partner for the day. Two counselors, not much older than my patient, gathered the necessary paperwork for an interagency transfer.

"She's all yours," said one.

"What's the problem?" I asked.

"She won't eat, says she is depressed and suicidal. She's also two months pregnant."

"How old is she?"

"Sixteen."

I took the papers and joined the girls in the truck. Andrea left the back to drive to Hasbro Children's Hospital, leaving me alone with a pregnant, sullen, suicidal sixteen-year-old. As the group home shrank from view through the rear windows, my patient visibly relaxed.

"What's going on?" I asked Alexandria.

"I'm hungry and they won't feed me. I'm eating for two and if my baby dies, I'm suing them. All I want is some candy. It's my candy and they won't let me have it. I can't eat the shit they call food. They want me to eat stinking round pizza. My boyfriend said he would bring ice cream but they won't let him. Them stupid bitches, I'm going to sue them and everybody they know if my baby dies."

"Besides that, what's going on?" I asked. She looked at me for the first time. She looked afraid.

"I don't want to stay there."

"How long have you been there?"

"Since Tuesday."

"Did you come from foster care or home?"

"Home. I want to go back."

The rescue stopped suddenly.

"What's going on?" I asked Andrea.

"I don't know but two motorcycle cops have shut down the highway. They're trying to rush us through."

Once we got past the barricade, Alexandria and I unbuckled our seat belts and hunched by the rear windows, trying to see what was going on.

"Slow down," I asked Andrea. She stopped the truck on the exit ramp. We all watched as a procession of state, local, and federal police drove past us. I'd never seen such an impressive procession.

"Who do you think it is?" Alexandria asked.

"I don't know, some big shot. Maybe the president. Andrea, back up a little, I want to see better," I shouted over my shoulder to the front.

"You can back up on the highway?" Alexandria asked, impressed now.

"Of course, we're Rescue 1. You don't mind, do you?"

"Hell no!" she answered.

Andrea backed up about one hundred feet so we could see better. After about thirty police cars and motorcycles, a hearse came into view. Alexandria asked if I knew who died. I didn't. I asked her if she knew who it was. She didn't. We watched the endless procession drive down Interstate 95.

"They're probably heading toward the Veterans Cemetery," I said. "My father is buried there too."

She just looked out the rear windows as we got going. I wondered what she was thinking. When I checked her in at the triage desk at Hasbro, I told the nurse her story, adding that although she was trouble at the group home, I found her to be rather pleasant.

"It's the culture," the nurse said. "She won't be very nice to me, I'm sure. I'll remind her of her mother."

I wonder if Alexandria has a father who cares. Maybe her situation wouldn't be so dire if there was a responsible man in her life.

Stay in Narragansett

Every time his girlfriend started to speak he yelled, "Shut up!" She was sobbing next to their car, a new BMW with considerable front-end damage. Dave, the lieutenant on Engine 7, stood to the side observing. The guy asked Dave something and Dave apparently didn't respond the way he liked.

Dave, not shy by any means, stood looking at the guy with his arms crossed. I was impressed with his restraint. The guy who crashed his car went on and on spewing some nonsense about how much he hates Providence, how we were a bunch of punks, and how he wished he was back in Narragansett with his $500,000 home. His girlfriend spoke up, trying to talk sense into the moron.

"Shut up," he screamed at her. Neither was hurt in the accident. I had her sign a refusal form, clearing the Providence Fire Department and myself from liability should the lovely couple from Narragansett sober up, consult their attorney, and decide to include us in their lawsuit. The guy was continuing his drivel about the morons who interrupted his perfect night by allowing him to crash his car into the bridge abutment at Memorial and College Streets.

I truly don't know how Dave refrained from clobbering this guy. I made one attempt to have him sign the refusal; he was behaving like a five-year-old. No problem. I wrote up the report, stated the intoxicated person refused to be treated or transported, and refused to sign the refusal. We left him with his girlfriend, the cops, and the tow truck. I hope his girlfriend smartens up before it is too late.

Saviors

The stairs were spongy, soft and dark. I used the Maglite Captain Healy gave me for Christmas to light the narrow passageway.

"I've never seen him like this," said a sixteen-year-old boy who led us up the stairway into the third-floor apartment. The place was clean, tiny, and barely furnished. The front room served as the boy's bedroom. A small cot occupied one corner, an old TV another. No big-screen, stereo, or fancy things, just bare necessities.

We walked through the kitchen toward the bedroom. There, a fiftyish man lay on his back, soaked with sweat. A bowl of uneaten pork was next to his bed, which was actually a twin mattress with clean sheets laying on the floor. The boy was a wreck.

"He won't answer me, he can't get up, I didn't know what to do," he said, concern for his dad obvious.

"Has he been drinking?" I asked.

"He had some E&J brandy," the boy told us. "But he doesn't get drunk. He's not a bum, he works seven days a week. He doesn't have any medical problems, no medications or allergies," he told us when asked.

The kid was near tears as he watched me and Jeff try to wake the guy up. It was six in the morning, my twenty-ninth run since I showed up for work thirty-seven hours ago. I honestly didn't think I would be able to carry him down the stairs to the rescue. The frustration having to cater to the endless flood of needless 911 calls takes its toll eventually.

Unfortunately, the people who need and deserve first-rate medical care delivered in a professional way are the ones who suffer when the people they called for help show up at their door exhausted and cynical. Thankfully, Jeff took over.

"I'll get the chair," he said and left the apartment. I tried again to wake up the patient enough so we could help him down the stairs. No luck. The guy was incapable. Jeff came back with the chair and set it up, the war of wills lost. Somehow I mustered the energy to carry the guy down the rickety, dark stairs and into the rescue. We did some vitals and found the problem. His glucose level was 34.

I told the kid what we were doing as we started the IV and administered an amp D-50 and 100 mg of thiamine. As the medication took effect, the patient improved considerably. The son held his father's hand as he regained consciousness. The simple act of kindness between father and son made me forget all the nonsense, the drunks, morons from Narragansett, and abuse.

To witness such an act of grace between two people I initially dismissed as just more work in an endless shift was the greatest gift I can remember receiving.

Sinking

"Do you have any idea when he took the pills?" I asked his son once we had the patient in the rescue.

"My aunt called around six and said I had better get home, something wasn't right," he replied. "Is he going to be okay?"

"He'll be fine," I said confidently. "Worse case scenario they'll have to pump his stomach."

I wanted to reassure the man's son, who was in his early twenties. They lived in a nice house in the Mount Pleasant section of the city. Pictures of Boston sports stars decorated the place, not much sign of a female presence.

"Has he ever done anything like this before?" I asked.

"Never. He drinks a little and has been depressed for a few weeks but he has been getting help. His girlfriend left him last month but he has been doing better."

"Are you coming with us?" I asked.

"I'll follow in my car."

"Why don't you meet us at the hospital, he'll be fine." I didn't want him following the rescue. Bad things tend to happen when people do that.

"Don't worry, take your time," I said, closing the rear doors of the rescue as he watched his father lie on the stretcher. The guys from Engine 15 were getting vital signs and starting an IV. The patient, who had walked with help from his house to the rescue, was now unconscious, BP 90/55 with a pulse of 110, pulsox 90 percent. His pupils were pinpoint, respirations shallow, 14 per minute.

"He's going downhill," I stated the obvious. I drew 2 mg of Narcan and had Henry push it through the IV line. It didn't do any good at all.

"I need a driver."

Jeff and I stayed in back while Henry drove toward Rhode Island Hospital with Engine 15 following. A seemingly routine call was going bad. Jeff got the bag-valve device set up while I drew two more milligrams of Narcan.

Another BP, 86/40. I looked at the bag of empty medication bottles. Tenormin, Coumadin, Klonopin, and Seroquel. The Narcan was ineffective, his respirations sinking and his BP dropping. I called RIH triage and gave them the report, ETA three minutes. There was nothing more I could do for now. I thought of getting the ET kit ready but didn't have time to intubate. I wish I hadn't been so nonchalant with his son.

At the hospital the medical team stood ready in Trauma Room 1. They gave more Narcan, assisted ventilations, then intubated. The man's son arrived as I was walking out. I didn't know what to say to him.

Huh?

She had a pain in the neck so she called 911.

"When did the pain begin?" I asked.

"About an hour after I got home from surgery."

"When was the surgery?"

"Yesterday."

"What was the surgery for?"

"Neck pain."

"Do you take any medications?"

"I have a prescription but I haven't filled it yet."

"What is the prescription for?"

"Pain."

Water

I was watching *Saving Private Ryan* when my phone rang. It was my brother, Bob, calling from Iraq. I hadn't heard from him in around two weeks. He was "on a mission."

We talked for a while, pretended things were normal for a few minutes. When that got old, we talked about his situation. Grim, he acknowledged. Not much more can be said, but grim. He misses his wife and kids. We miss him. He's back at his base, the plywood walls of his quarters welcome after two weeks on the road. Baghdad is especially disturbing, he said. Two weeks through hell to transport water.

When I hung up I tried to watch the rest of the movie. When we were kids we would spend Saturday afternoons watching war movies on an old TV in our basement. I must be getting old and soft; I could barely focus on the screen through my blurred vision.

I wiped my eyes with my sleeve and turned the TV off.

Game Over

"Think he'll mind if we change the channel?"

"He's dead."

"It doesn't feel right."

"It is the AFC Championship."

"Right."

"I don't want to touch the TV, it's all sticky."

"How do you know, you haven't touched it."

"You've got gloves on."

"I'll do it."

We watched the end of the second half with a dead thirty-year-old guy. He was shirtless, kneeling with his swollen purple face pressed against the filthy linoleum. Cockroaches watched us from the ceiling as we waited for a police sergeant to clear the scene. An empty syringe lay on a bureau, next to a hot plate. His last meal sat at the bottom of the pan, rice, beans, and roaches, hours old. We forgot about the dead guy and focused on the game. My skin was crawling when the sergeant showed up. I told him my time on scene, now officially the time of death, and left.

Too Late?

"Yeah, and I'm a rookie."

"I'm telling you, I didn't do any heroin."

"What are these?" I held up four syringes filled with a murky brown liquid.

"Heroin, but I didn't do any."

"Why are your pupils pinpoints?"

"I've been smoking crack since yesterday." He held up a rock and a glass pipe as proof.

"What's the heroin for?"

"In case I need to calm down."

"This much will probably kill you."

"I wasn't going to do it all at once."

I emptied the syringes and disposed of the sharps. He sat on the bench seat as we rode to Rhode Island Hospital. I couldn't leave him to drive the car we found him in so we left it in a hotel parking lot. He fidgeted as we drove; I asked him what the hell he was doing.

"I was clean for seven months, had a fight with my girlfriend a couple of days ago and kind of lost my mind."

"You're going to be back on the streets in a few hours. Why don't you get yourself to an NA meeting before it's too late."

"It's already too late."

"It's never too late."

We walked into the ER together. I hope he takes my advice and gets back on track and doesn't smoke the crack I forgot to take away from him.

Appreciation

He thought it was all his fault. His wife was on the stretcher, cervical collar in place and lying immobilized on the long backboard. Shattered glass covered her coat, mixed with spatters of blood, magnifying the effect. She was dazed but not critical. Her husband, injured himself, refused to be treated. He needed to take care of his wife. I understood.

They held hands in back of the rescue. He was getting in the way so we worked around him. Blood pressure first, some oxygen, an IV. I shined my light into her eyes and saw her pupils react properly. The three-inch laceration on the back of her head had been treated by John, from Engine 7. I'm sure he has seen much worse during his deployment in Iraq at the start of the war, though he never says much about it.

The ride to Rhode Island Hospital was short. The accident happened on I-95 in front of the exit ramp to the ER. My guess is somebody in a pickup truck missed the exit, stopped in the travel lane to back up, and was struck by the couple now in my rescue. They never had a chance. I told the man he did a great job avoiding what could and should have been two fatalities. He continued to blame himself, thinking he should have been able to avoid the truck.

They had been driving to their home in Coventry, about ten miles down the highway, when everything stopped. He told me his wife screamed "Look out," and he only had an instant to react. An eighteen-wheeler was on his right, another car on his left. He did all he could do.

His midsized car crashed into the back of the pickup on an angle toward the right front side. Had he swerved into the eighteen-wheeler, they would have been crushed. Had he swerved into the other car, they probably would have spun out and rolled over. In my fifteen years on the fire department, I have seen a lot of people killed in the exact spot their accident occurred.

Perhaps these two were lucky; maybe fate was on their side. I say the guy reacted perfectly in a bad situation and saved his wife's life.

"Get off the cross, we need the wood," I told him as we backed into the rescue bay at the ER.

Throughout the night and into the next morning I talked to the man. His wife was out of the trauma room and in critical care. Every time I brought another patient in, our paths would cross. He couldn't thank me enough. I told him I didn't do anything anybody else would have done but he refused to believe me.

"You did what they would do," he said, "but you put all of your heart into it." He introduced me to his family who straggled in as the long night went on. I was a bit embarrassed by the attention.

I would be lying if I said I didn't appreciate it.

Sisters

Sister One left her three kids with Sister Two and went to Boston to stay with her boyfriend for the week. On Friday night she decided she wanted her kids with her. After partying for a while she showed up at Sister Two's house, drunk. The kids and Sister Two were not there. They were in Olneyville; Sister Two wanted to give the kids a treat, so she rounded them up and went to get wieners at two thirty in the morning. When Sister One found her kids missing she got mad. Really mad. When Sister Two came back at three in the morning with the kids, Sister One attacked her, stabbing her in the face five times. The cops were called but Sister Two didn't press charges, so they sent the kids home with Sister One. Sister Two called 911 for a rescue.

That is where I came into the fray.

When I showed up, Sister One was gone with the kids and Sister Two was waiting for us on her front steps. Her wounds were not life threatening but would leave scars. She had a puncture wound under her nose on the left side of her face, one under her lip on the right side, another two on her forehead, and one on top of her head for good measure. She ranted and raved about the bitch that is her sister as we rode to the ER. I only heard Sister Two's story. I'm sure Sister One sees things completely differently. I'm also sure that the kids have seen too much already.

Thirty Years

I've been playing guitars since I was fourteen. I've almost got the Aerosmith song "Same Old Song and Dance" down. It was the first song I tried to learn, and I've been working on it for thirty years.

One day at the station, my friend Jeff asked me to teach him a few chords. I showed him some easy ones: D, C, Am, G.

"Learn those and get back to me," I said, then forgot about it.

Last week, I was trying to learn a Foo Fighters song, "Times Like These." The chords looked pretty easy. Days into it, Jeff came into my office.

"You might be able to play this," I said to him, thinking it would be difficult but not impossible for him to play. He picked up my guitar and went to the dorm. Less than an hour later he returned, sat down and played the song, start to finish, and sang the verses.

The best I can do is hum along to "Wild Thing" while switching two chords. I wanted to throw the guitar out the window. Thirty years is a long time. When I got home I went to my basement, plugged in, and let some hideous noise loose from my Ibanez Les Paul (lawsuit model 1976).

Thirty years, three chords. Rock on!

CHAPTER 6
FEBRUARY

Sleep Tight

The city is lively tonight, the usual suspects drunk and helpless providing a steady stream of 911 calls. Toby Keith is playing to a sold-out Dunk. The "granny drop" has been in full swing since this morning. Super Bowl Sunday and all, no room for sick old people at home. Diabetics, seizures, MVAs, and all that go with it have filled the area hospitals.

I don't know if we need more hospitals or less sick people. I do know that the people we have need to find a better way to take care of themselves. I often wonder what would happen if a true large-scale emergency happened. We survived the Station fire thanks to the heroic deeds of the people who worked that horrific night. That was one incident involving four hundred people and it nearly crippled the system. I hope to never find out how we could treat thousands.

No Delivery!

The house was dark and locked up tight. Somewhere inside a full-term maternity waited. Captain Healy directed his guys to find a way in. A window turned out to be the best way, they forced it without damage, Vicro and Ralph crawled through and opened the door. We heard someone moaning at the top of the stairs; a woman named Lovely, nine months pregnant, due today with constant contractions.

"I feel like my belly is going to explode!" she said as we put her into the stair chair and carried her out the door of her apartment and into the rescue. I had a bulb syringe and clamps ready, the blanket and a catcher's mitt sat on the bench next to the stretcher. Renato started an IV as we sped toward Women and Infants Hospital. Steve stayed in back with us to help with the delivery. It was a five-minute ride.

"Is she crowning?" I asked Steve as I filled out the report from the captain's seat. He opened his eyes wide, shook his head, and took a look. The contractions were constant, her water had broken, delivery imminent. Three minutes to the delivery room.

"Don't push!" Lovely was a trooper but a very loud one. The contractions continued but no crowning. Her blood pressure was 178/120. Two minutes away. I called the triage desk at W&I and gave my report.

"Twenty-seven-year-old pregnant female, due today, constant contractions, two minutes away."

Nothing much to do now but wait and hope we got to the hospital in time. In fifteen years I have never delivered a baby. I want to keep it that way. I've read all there is to read in the books but am petrified of it actually happening. Firefighters and EMTs deliver babies all the time. It's one of the best experiences one can have, I've heard. The mother does all the work; unless there are complications things take care of themselves, I've heard.

We arrived at the ER, no delivery. Lovely was fully dilated and taken "upstairs." She delivered as we were walking back to the truck.

My record is intact.

Winter

I wonder why he was outside on an eight-degree night, dressed in jeans and a short-sleeve T-shirt with only a down vest to protect him from the elements. The wind chill was well below zero. If he had a destination in mind he never made it. Somebody saw a crumpled heap lying on the sidewalk and called 911.

He was conscious; barely. No ID in any of his pockets and he couldn't tell us his name. We found him at 5:00 a.m. Another hour and he would have been dead. He'll probably lose the fingers on his right hand from frostbite, the left ones have a chance. Cocaine and barbiturates were found in his blood. This has been a mild winter for most of us but a cruel one for the guy we found frozen to the sidewalk.

Emily

Four adults had her pinned to the floor, each holding a limb. Her foster mother stood to the side shaking her head.

"She'll be like this for hours," she said. The guys from Engine 12 stood back and waited for some direction. We are not trained or authorized to use restraints. The patient, a ten-year-old deaf girl named Emily, continued to struggle as we figured out what to do.

"How do I say her name?" I asked one of the people in the room, a teacher at the Rhode Island School for the Deaf. He showed me. I formed my hand into a representation of the letter E, then bumped my chin with it twice.

"How do I say my name?" I asked. I bumped my M-shaped hand to my chin twice and knelt beside her.

"Tell her we have to put her on our bed and take her to the hospital." The teacher signed the message, Emily responded. She said she would go only if the firefighters went with her.

"She spits," somebody said. I decided to put a surgical mask on her.

"She'll gnaw on it and might choke. The last time they put masks on themselves," said the mother.

There was no way a beautiful, scared ten-year-old was going to make us wear masks. I put the mask on my face, looked at Emily, pointed to her, then the mask. She understood and shook her head, yes. Without a whimper, she let me place the mask over her face, never losing eye contact. I had the guys take over holding her and lifted her to the stretcher. My grip on her arm relaxed as she relaxed. Before I knew it I was just holding her hand as she stopped struggling. We let her go. The staff at the school were impressed, but I'm pretty sure Emily was plain out of gas. She pointed at her backpack as we wheeled her into the corridor. One of the firefighters from Engine 12, Dave, handed it to her. He was as captivated by her as I was. She reached inside and took out a little electronic video game and started to play.

Inside the rescue, Dave kept her entertained while I filled out the report. She was fascinated by everything. She wanted us to take her blood pressure and pulsox so we did. She pointed at the heart monitor. We ran an EKG. She knew which button to push for a printout. I let the paper roll. She folded it neatly and stashed it inside her backpack. Emily's smile lit the back of the rescue.

At the hospital we waited for her foster mom and the interpreter from the school. Emily sat on the stretcher and played with me and Dave. Her hair was a mess, her skin still red from the exertion, and her brilliant blue eyes still swollen from crying, but still she was beautiful. We put her on the hospital stretcher without any trouble as the mom and interpreter came in. As we wheeled her into one of the treatment rooms, I asked the mom about the tantrums.

"She was good for a while but I've had to leave work three times this month," she said.

"What causes them?" I asked.

"She has been through a lot. Her mother was making money using her. Her father is in prison for the same thing." I heard her but didn't comprehend. "She was being prostituted."

As they wheeled Emily away, she looked over her shoulder at me and Dave, gave us a big smile and a wave. I watched until they turned the corner and disappeared. Dave didn't hear about her past. I considered telling him but decided not to burden him. Instead I walked outside into the bright sunshine, found a quiet spot, and sat there until the cold air made me numb.

Come Home
Somebody was waiting at home.

Midnight, twelve thirty. One.

They must have been frantic. A phone call shattering the silence, one nobody should have to hear. "There has been an accident."

A truck hauling scrap metal was traveling south on 95. Interstate 95 splits into 195 from the left-hand lanes, confusing even for people familiar with the roadway as you roll through Providence. The trucker from Gettysburg, Pennsylvania, was in the wrong lane. When he realized his mistake and tried to veer right back onto 95, his load shifted and the truck tipped onto its side, crushing the car in the next lane. A woman was driving home. She never made it.

The scene was chaos as firefighters tried desperately to clear the sharp metal from the overturned truck. A hole was cut into the roof to expedite things. As I walked the injured truck driver past the horrific sight, he stopped and looked, visibly shaken by the sight. The rear tire was all we could see of the car crushed beneath the truck. At that point we didn't know how many were in the car. It could have been full of kids.

When enough debris was cleared, Zack Kenyon, the lieutenant from Rescue 4, crawled through and assessed the situation. One victim, female, fifties, no pulse, deformities, deceased.

Renato and I transported the trucker to Rhode Island Hospital. He had been driving trucks without incident for thirty years. He wanted to call his wife back home but his cell phone was lost in the debris.

When I got back to the station I called Cheryl. She yelled at me for calling so late. The sound of her voice was bittersweet.

In Our Midst
A man dies in a heroic attempt at saving his daughter's life. Time and time again he tries, stopping only when he has nothing left to give. His teenage daughter clings to life, third-degree burns over 60 percent of her body, scarred for life, however long that may be. A mother and son face an uncertain future, heartache, loss, and economic disaster. Firefighters battle the early morning blaze, fearless warriors protecting the lives and property of the citizens of Providence.

Outside the inferno, two firefighters wait, detailed to Rescue 6 for the night. One from a ladder truck, the other from an engine company. They watch, knowing they should be inside with their brothers doing what they do best, fighting fire. The pulseless, burned body of the teenage girl is brought to them from the charred ruin. With minimal rescue experience in an unfamiliar setting, they do their job better than anybody has the right to expect. This incident and countless others get a small mention for a day on the local news, an article in the local section of the paper, until something more lurid comes along.

Everywhere I look I see images of Anna Nicole Smith. Her tragic end is on the front page in the newspapers nationwide, lead story on network stations, twenty-four hours on CNN,

MSNBC, and FOX. The media panders to a society that lives with heroes and superstars right in their midst. Our soldiers die fighting a war that has lost its luster with the media. Without "in-depth coverage," paparazzi, or fanfare, we walk side by side with greatness, regular citizens as important and newsworthy as the "stars."

Some of us make our living where our mettle is put to the test daily. Others go about their business until tragedy strikes, and then find within themselves the courage and conviction to make a difference.

Then there are those who are fascinated by the glamorous images projected in front of them as they live their lives in front of their TV screen, waiting for somebody to save them.

Close Call

The Rescue Gods are toying with me. A twenty-one-year-old called with contractions two minutes apart. We were three minutes away from the hospital. Water broke, patient screamed, I broke out the catcher's mitt. We arrived at Women and Infants at 0008 hours. A baby boy was born at 0009 hours. This one never made it upstairs. She barely made it off my stretcher. My record is still intact, barely. I have tempted fate; it's only a matter of time now. I may have to make a sacrifice to appease the gods. Maybe I'll let the next one push and get it over with.

Breathe

As the night wore on his lungs filled with fluid. Finally, his wife called 911. When we arrived he was struggling for air, diaphoretic and nearly unconscious. His vitals showed his pulsox at 83 percent, BP 220/148, respirations around 40 with a heart rate of 140.

At a fit seventy-five years old, Daniel looked like he could have been most of the guys' grandfather or, in some of our cases, father. With help from Engine 12 we carried him to the rescue. Renato started an IV, Issac set up the O_2 with an albuterol treatment, I slipped a nitro tab under his tongue. I could see fear in Daniel's eyes as he labored for every breath.

He had a history of congestive heart failure. His wife gave me his medication list on the way out the door. I saw aspirin and Lasix on the list. I filled a syringe with double his daily dose of Lasix and pushed it through the IV line. For me, one of the most gratifying moments of the job is seeing the effects of our work evident on the face of the people we help. Within minutes the albuterol started to help clear his lungs, blood flow was increased by the nitro, the Lasix helped pass fluid from his lungs, and the oxygen helped considerably.

I reassessed his vital signs. Pulsox, 96 percent, BP 168/110, respirations 24 with a pulse of 110. Not bad. The best vital sign was the look of relief that showed on his rugged face. We transported him to Our Lady of Fatima Hospital. He was able to say thank you and shake our hands as we left. I thought to myself as we rode back to the station as the sun was rising how fortunate I am to have this job.

Ice Rescue Drill

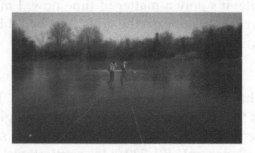

Drew and Seth from Engine 11 cut a hole in the ice. One went into the freezing water, the other one rescued him. They switched places and did it again. Division 1, Battalion 2,

Special Hazards, Ladder 5, Engine 13, Engine 10, and Rescue 1 took part in the drill organized by Lieutenant Grantham of Engine 11. His guys did a great job.

Risk Taking

He appeared a lot more dazed than he should have. The damage to his Camry was minor. The pickup he hit had only a scratch and a broken taillight. The guys from Engine 10 saw something wasn't right.

"He might have had a stroke," said Bruce as we tried to get him to tell us what happened.

"I can't move my left arm," he said, speech slurred. I didn't think he was intoxicated. We rolled the stretcher to the driver's door and lifted him onto it. The frozen rain and sleet that had been falling for most of the day and previous night made the footing treacherous and soaked us and the patient, a sixty-one-year-old guy from Cranston, as we worked.

In back the situation came clear. Brad, my partner for the day, was working overtime. He started an IV while I got the patients vitals. BP 212/140, pulse 74, pulsox 96 percent with a glucose level of 110. He had a facial droop on his left side along with left-sided weakness. Probable CVA. We hooked him up with high-flow oxygen, applied a cervical collar and ran an EKG, then started toward Rhode Island Hospital. I was able to get some answers as we sped toward the ER.

He had been shoveling snow when he felt weak on his left side. He waited for half an hour for the feeling to go away. When it got worse, he got into his car and started to drive himself to the hospital. Sometimes the people who need us most don't want to "bother" us.

"Why didn't you call 911?" I asked him.

"I figured you guys were busy with real emergencies," he said.

At the hospital the doctors confirmed our findings. He was a candidate for an aggressive but risky treatment for stroke patients. The treatment has something to do with thinning the blood. When it works, loss of function is minimal. He was having a major stroke and tried to drive himself to the hospital. My guess is he will decide to take the chance.

Real Trouble
"He looks pretty big," said Don Touro as we approached the crowd.

"He'll be alright, I've had him before."

Jonathan stood with a Providence cop and the guys from Engine 10, holding his bruised and bloodied hand.

"What happened?"

"He was mad and punched the walls at his group home," Lieutenant Deedy from Engine 10 told me. "It doesn't look too bad."

As Don Touro bandaged the damaged hand, Jonathan told me what happened.

"The people at the group home keep telling me I won't be nothin' when I get out of here. I'm going to be eighteen next month and on my own. They said I'm not ready but Carcieri is lettin' all the eighteen-year-olds loose."

In an effort to trim the Rhode Island state budget, Governor Carcieri has proposed drastic cuts to social programs. Among them is a provision releasing patients under the care of the Department of Children, Youth, and Families at age eighteen as opposed to the current cutoff age of twenty-one. When I read about it in the paper and heard it on the news, it sounded like a great idea. Decisions affecting other people are easy to make from the comfort of home.

"Why were you punching the walls?" I asked Jonathan as we rode toward Hasbro Children's Hospital.

"I just get mad and lose it," he said. "I told the counselor that said I was never going to make it I was going to kill her. Then I punched the window but it wouldn't break so I went outside and threw rocks at it but I kept missing. I ran a few streets away and started punching a brick wall. Then the cops came, then you came, and here we are."

He is a big seventeen-year-old kid with a lot of problems. He has been in group homes since he was four and heavily medicated. This wasn't the first time I took him to the hospital because of his outbursts. I don't know if the group home is the answer, but I do know that if they set him loose next month he will be in real trouble.

CHAPTER 7
MARCH

Hard Times

He sat on the cold street holding his foot in his hands. It was still attached to his leg, but barely. I winced every time he tried to put it back where it belonged. With help from the crew of Engine 8 we loaded him into the rescue. I left the boot on but cut off the pant leg, exposing the bloody sock and compound fracture.

Jorge was conscious; he looked more upset than anything. We held him still, started an IV, and transported him to Rhode Island Hospital. No pain medication—Rescue 6 does without morphine.

Jorge had no ID, no home, and now no livelihood. His immigration status is most likely illegal. How quickly things change. He was fortunate his injury didn't happen in Guatemala—his leg would probably be gone. It will be months, if ever, before he walks again. His injury will cost the system tens of thousands of dollars. He came here for the work, probably sending most of his earnings home. He and his family have some hard times ahead.

Elvis

All she had was a wheelchair, a couch, a bed, and a picture of Elvis. The place was clean; when you don't have anything it's easy to keep up. From her bed she told us about her pain.

"Four days now, getting worse every day."

Living with diabetes for twenty of her fifty-three years had taken its toll. What little I recall of my grandmother's mother is an old lady in a wheelchair with no legs. She lost them to the "sugar" was all I was told.

We brought her to the truck, got her comfortable, and headed toward Rhode Island Hospital. It was a long transport for us, about twelve minutes. I settled into the captain's chair and started the report while "Louise" sobbed in the stretcher. It was a busy night, the radio blared in the back.

"Rescue 2 and Engine 14 to Manton Avenue for difficulty breathing."

"Rescue 5 and Engine 7 to Benefit Street for a man who has fallen."

"Rescue 4 to 100 Broad Street in the lobby for an intoxicated male."

"Engine 4 with an East Providence Rescue to Blackstone Boulevard for chest pains."

And on and on.

I turned the volume all the way down. From the cab came a familiar sound.

"A little Elvis for your listening pleasure," Jeff yelled back as we rolled down the highway. "Don't Be Cruel," "Hound Dog," then "Teddy Bear." Louise sat up in the stretcher, stopped sobbing, and actually smiled. It was the best ride of the night. Sometimes Jeff's music is the perfect medicine.

Norman

He's not sick, not stupid, and not homeless. When he is tired, or cold, or hungry, he'll call 911 and say his legs hurt, or he is bleeding rectally, or he has abdominal pain. We take him to the ER, they treat him, and he is shown the door. He walks to the nearest pay phone, and with discharge papers in one hand and the phone in the other he calls 911 for a ride to a different hospital.

At restaurants he eats a full-course dinner, clutches his chest, and yells for somebody to call 911. Of course, somebody does, we show up and take him to the hospital. The restaurant eats the tab, the servers go without a gratuity, the "patient" wins again.

He is a heavy man, fifty years old and diabolical. Time and time again we give him the lecture. Somebody could die while he abuses the system, a kid could be choking, heart attacks, accidents, and he could care less. He is getting his. I have never seen anybody with such absolute disregard for his fellow man.

Our system of government is the most successful civilization has ever seen. The Constitution is a brilliant document giving us all the rights afforded within, most importantly the right to pursue our own happiness. People like Norman, if allowed, will crush our pursuit of happiness. The legal system that is based on the Constitution has been corrupted to the point where it would no longer be recognizable to the people who wrote it.

Norman and thousands like him are allowed to exist and make a mockery of our laws by the very people who are educated and trained to uphold the laws but have chosen to corrupt them instead.

Lawyers
If I were to leave Norman at the pay phone, or if the police were to arrest him at the restaurants where he is having his alleged chest pain, or if we or the hospitals refused to treat him and in the unlikely event he actually had a real emergency,

there would be a trainload of them waiting to fill their pockets. The fact that people like Norman are allowed to thrive among us makes me wonder if we can ever get ourselves back on track. I certainly hope so. Until then, I'll take Norman the two blocks back to the hospital when he calls.

Or maybe not.

Rescue

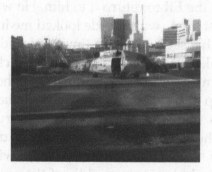

He was hauling lobster pots up from the bottom of the ocean, eighty miles off Nantucket, when he lost three of his fingers. His shipmates packed the severed digits in ice, wrapped them in plastic, and gave them to him. He put them into the top pocket of his coat. The captain radioed for help. The Coast Guard sent a rescue helicopter. The fishermen waited on the freezing ocean for help to arrive.

We got the patient out of the helicopter and into the rescue without much fuss. He was a tough-looking Spanish-speaking guy, his left hand wrapped with gauze and duct tape. The crew of the fishing vessel did a great job with what they had. The flight nurse came with us to give the report to the staff at the ER. He was a young, good-looking guy, dressed in his orange jumpsuit. With his rescue gear he looked pretty impressive. When we arrived at the ER,

Teresa, the lieutenant in charge of Rescue 5, opened the rear doors and told him she liked his outfit. The flight nurse was very impressed with her, as any guy in his right mind would be. We got the patient through the triage desk and into the treatment area.

We took the Coast Guard guy back to the chopper. They took off toward their base, we were heading back to our station when I saw the fisherman's life vest on the floor of the rescue. There was some expensive-looking gear on it, so I went back to the ER to return it to him. He was sitting on a stretcher in fast track, waiting. He looked me in the eye, held my gaze for what seemed a long time, and said, "Thank you, señor." He looked at his disfigured hand and closed his eyes.

This was my last run of a thirty-four-hour shift. No sleep, nonstop calls. Instead of feeling exhausted, I was exhilarated. A man can come to this country, find honest work, live without fear and pursue whatever dreams he has. When tragedy strikes there are people who will scramble to a helicopter, find him in the middle of the ocean, fly him to a hospital, put him in a rescue where a beautiful lieutenant opens the door for him, be treated with care, kindness, and respect, and be given the best medical treatment in the world. No questions asked, no thanks necessary, just a country full of people willing and trained to help. It makes me proud to be an American citizen.

Tough Job
She handed me a license and registration. I gave it a quick look before getting her and her friend into the truck. Their car had moderate damage to the rear end; whoever hit them hit them hard from the look of things. I looked at the pile of debris scattered on the street, searching for some clue as to the identity of the owner of the hit-and-run vehicle but there

was nothing but broken glass and plastic. Sometimes, if we are lucky, the license plate falls off. Not this time.

Renato had things well in hand when I returned to the truck. Our two victims were in cervical collars and lying on backboards.

"Did you get the license plate number?" I asked.

"No, but you shouldn't need it," said the passenger, an eighteen-year-old girl from Smithfield.

"Why not?" I asked. The driver, another eighteen-year-old girl from Smithfield, looked up from the stretcher.

"You have her license and registration in your hand."

The girls had been out dancing at one of the downtown clubs. They looked like they belonged in a music video rather than on a backboard in a Providence rescue. They were in good spirits, all things considered. Their injuries were minor, their car probably fixable. A police officer came to the side door.

"The driver of the hit and run gave them this before she left the scene," I said, handing the license and registration of the suspect over to him. He looked at me, the girls, and the evidence in his hand.

It's a tough job, but somebody has to do it.

Fresh Air

For days she sat on her couch in her filthy apartment, struggling to breathe. At three in the morning she called.

Trouble breathing. Her O_2 tank and mask lay at her feet.

"Why aren't you using your oxygen?"

"I can't breathe."

"That is what the oxygen is for."

"Help me."

"Help yourself," I said and put her oxygen mask back on. Twenty prescription bottles sat on her coffee table next to a remote control. Oxygen tubing was tangled everywhere; I'm amazed she never strangled herself. Andy and I carried all three hundred pounds of her down three flights of narrow stairs into the freezing night air. Getting out of the house and leaving her cigarettes behind did her a world of good.

Over There

Hector is back in charge of Rescue 2. He doesn't look any different but I'm sure his time in Iraq has changed him in ways we will never see. Those closest to him may notice the subtle changes, the rest of us are happy just to have him home. As the War on Terror grinds on and public opinion turns sour, our soldiers continue to fight, continue to die.

Nine more yesterday.

Every person serving our country in Iraq and Afghanistan has something in common. The people they leave behind jump at the opportunity to let anyone and everyone know that their brother, son, daughter, mother, friend, uncle, neighbor, or even the guy at work they normally mumble a good morning to is there, in harms way. It makes us feel special, as though just knowing somebody "over there" puts us on a higher level.

My brother, Bob, is still in Iraq. He's about halfway through his deployment. Whenever the war is mentioned, I stand a little taller and tell anybody who will listen, "My brother is there!"

Thanks, Bob. Thanks, Hector. Thanks to everybody "over there."

Melting (EMS 1 essay winner, EMS Week, 2009)

I knew I was the minority before walking into the restaurant. It's something I have gotten used to. Good food smells the same to everybody. I had no idea what they were selling but I couldn't wait to take a bite. A group of men sat in a booth speaking a language that has become familiar, yet hard for me to understand. They looked in my direction, then returned to their conversation.

The restaurant is set up cafeteria style, all the offerings displayed on steam tables or in refrigerated cases. I placed my order with the girl behind the counter, certain it would be delicious. It was. When I paid I thanked the girl in her language. Her smile transformed her face from pretty to beautiful. She returned the thanks and still smiled as I left. The guys watched me leave.

Years ago I began working in this area. I have seen many changes. At first I felt like an outsider; it was obvious that I didn't belong here. I was treated differently from the people who lived in the neighborhood. They seemed to tolerate my presence, but patiently waited for me to go.

Whether these thoughts were real or imagined I will never know. I do know that I no longer feel that way. We have both changed, the neighborhood more diverse, myself accepting the way of the people who live and work here. Time has marched on and we have learned from and accepted our differences.

Riding through the neighborhood I marveled at the businesses that have replaced the abandoned buildings. Restaurants and grocery stores, beauty parlors, barbershops, nightclubs, delis, and boutiques are some examples of what the main street has to offer. Some mornings I see sidewalks being swept by proud business owners. In the afternoons shoppers fill the streets and stores. There are sidewalk vendors, food carts, and kids running everywhere. On weekend nights the dance clubs are full of people partying. They come from all over. The hardworking people out for a night of fun outnumber those looking for fights and trouble.

When I first came to this area, it was a dangerous place. The people on the street were to be avoided. Crime was prevalent, despair evident in the look of the people who lived here. Unfortunately, that element still exists. The difference is they are now the minority. People are free to go about their business with less trepidation. Danger lurks, but the cowards that prey on the ambitious have been forced into hiding. The good people outnumber the bad.

Progress is measured in many different ways. For years the city of Providence has been touted as the "Renaissance" city. Downtown enjoys an almost magical transformation. The streets are clean, business is booming, and economic development is evident throughout the area. All one has to do is look at the place and see it is on the verge of greatness. Guarded optimism abounds in the most jaded pessimist.

Hard work, faith, and perseverance have turned some of the city's most notorious neighborhoods into safe, lively destinations. Broadway, Westminster Street, and the West End all are reaping the rewards of deserved good press. People made this transformation possible, not politics. Honest, hardworking people have a way of finding the louts and getting rid of them. It takes time, but somehow, good prevails.

Downtown and the neighborhoods are on the way toward reaching their potential. This neighborhood is on a similar path; the essential ingredients are in place. I have gotten to know and respect many of the people here. Unfortunately, deadbeats abound. Some people will go to great lengths to avoid work. Government policies and generous social programs make it possible for struggling people to start climbing the social and economic ladder. These policies, designed and implemented to help struggling people get a foothold, have become corrupt. A culture exists which exploits the generosity of this country. I often encounter the attitude, "What can you do for me?" There are those that have to be carried by the rest of us. They appear to be beating the system, but by not participating in the work that makes this country great they are beating themselves. It is my hope that the progress made by the people making this neighborhood work is contagious. Every person has a stake in our future. Together, we can make it great.

I enjoy thinking about the past and future. I spend a lot of time driving through the different neighborhoods in this city. I look at the buildings and people, thinking of what was and what is to become. My great-grandparents came to this country from Sweden and Ireland. They settled in the area, and some worked as carpenters and helped build a lot of the homes that line these streets. They raised their families through tough times, but never lost their hope or drive. Their hard work set the foundation for future generations. I will always be inspired by and thankful for their sacrifice.

As I travel through Federal Hill, I reflect on another group of immigrant workers who came to this area with little more than a desire to prosper in their adopted land. Their language was foreign, their foods different. They were probably leery of the people who invaded their "turf." As years and generations passed, their place in the American culture solidified, became mainstream. Now, people from all over frequent the "Hill." Some of the words spoken by these immigrants in their native language have become a part of America's vernacular. People of all nationalities have a nostalgic feeling when they hear these words. It took some time, but their neighborhood "melted" into the "pot."

As I drive down Broad Street and look to the future I envision much the same.

My Gang
Beautiful day, sixty degrees. Looks like spring is here. I fired up the Yamaha V Star Bob is letting me use until he gets back from Iraq. It runs a little better than the '82 Honda CB900C I've been riding.

Last July, when the busload of soldiers from the 1207th was leaving Camp Fogarty, I took the old Honda to join in the farewell ceremonies. I noticed about fifty bikes lined up in front of and behind the buses. I asked one of the guys what was going on. He told me about his organization, the Patriot Guard, and invited me to join the procession. It was my first time in an actual motorcycle gang. I revved the engine and joined the other bikers at the back of the buses, pulling the old 900 right into the thick of things.

When the ceremonies were over and all the good-byes, hugs, and kisses exhausted, the 1207th boarded the buses amid cheers from the crowd of family, friends, and well-wishers. And of course the roar of fifty bikes, ready to roll. I sat among them, the roar deafening, the vibration of the bikes all around me. Finally, it was time to go. I released the clutch, gave the throttle some gas, and . . . nothing.

The other bikes stormed around me as I sat, trying to get her started. I saw the buses leave, the bikes in front and behind. When things quieted down I realized my bike had never started in the first place. The battery was dead. I needed a hill to get it push started that morning but thought the battery would have charged during the fifteen-mile ride to Fogarty. No such luck. My gang left me in the dust.

As the crowd left I sat by myself until Mary and Catherine came to my rescue. They were amused by my plight, and I was happy to take their minds off the departure of their husband and father. I was the least of their worries, but at least they got a chuckle on such a sad day. When all was clear I pushed the bike to a small decline where I mercifully was able to get it going. I never found my gang; they finished at the airport. I rode by as everybody was leaving.

Battling the Elements

"Rescue 1, respond to Chalkstone Avenue for a woman with a swollen hand."

"Rescue 1, responding."

A late season snowstorm was raging, traffic snarled all over the state. Renato was working overtime on Engine 15, near where this call originated. Whoever he was to relieve just lost two hours because we wouldn't be back for a while. We tried to get onto the highway but a gasoline tanker was stuck on the ramp. Somehow we maneuvered around it. I don't know how Renato did it; I closed my eyes during the whole thing. We crawled to our destination, a house in the Mount Pleasant section of the city, two blocks away from Roger Williams Medical Center. Fifteen minutes into our response, fire alarm contacted us to check on our progress.

"Delayed response, we're on Atwells, ETA ten minutes."

They dispatched an engine company to babysit while we crawled along, passing accidents and other mayhem. Our patient waited.

Eventually we arrived. The patient, a forty-four-year-old Spanish-speaking lady, had been shoveling snow when pain appeared on a finger on her left hand. It started to swell. She called 911. The swelling was gone when we got there, but she wanted—check that— insisted on being seen at the hospital. Not the hospital at the top of her street; she wanted Miriam Hospital, miles away.

Five thirty, Friday rush hour, raging snowstorm.

She had three firefighters from Engine 15 and two EMT/ firefighters from Rescue 1 to cater to her, yet she still was not satisfied. Her family was going to meet her at Miriam; that was where she needed to go.

"Your family should have stopped here and picked you up before meeting you at Miriam," I said.

She didn't, and probably never will understand.

Holding On

"Ladder 2 to fire alarm, advise Rescue 6 we have a fifty-year-old male, semiconscious, possible CHF, with a language barrier."

"Rescue 6 received."

Ryan pulled the rescue behind Ladder 2. He got the stair chair from the rear compartment and I made my way up the snow-covered steps into the first floor of the three-decker. Any thoughts of communicating with the patient and his family with my *Sesame Street* Spanish were forgotten as soon as I got near the door. Incense, probably jasmine, wafted through the doorway into the crisp morning air, a sure sign of an Asian family inside. Captain Varone met me at the door and gave me a brief rundown.

"He was okay at five this morning, then his wife found him like this. From what I can tell he has no prior medical conditions. They're looking for his medications now."

Our patient was on his back on the living room floor. His family, ten folks at least, crowded around, not knowing quite what to do, trusting us with their loved one's life. It is a responsibility that used to overwhelm me, but now I am honored by their trust. Carl, a firefighter from Ladder 2 with extensive rescue experience, was on his knees next to the man getting vital signs.

"It sounds like CHF," he said while listening through the stethoscope as the patient struggled to breathe. "110/58, pulse 90."

Ryan got the chair set up and we got ready to roll. We had him in the truck in about a minute, his family watching helplessly as we wheeled him out the door. Garrett drove the rescue, Jeff and the captain followed in the tower ladder. Ryan established an IV, Carl ran an EKG, and I contacted Rhode Island Hospital, telling them to get a medical team ready, ETA three minutes. A Cambodian girl who spoke English arrived just before we left and rode in the front, supplying information as we worked.

The man on the stretcher stopped breathing about a minute into the transport. Ryan had the bag-valve mask ready and started to assist ventilations. I slipped a nitro tab under his tongue and pushed 80 mg of Lasix, hoping to help him breathe. As we pulled into the ER he began to breathe on his own and opened his eyes. The medical team was ready in Trauma Room 1. I gave them what I knew.

"Fifty-three-year-old male, last seen conscious by family at five this morning, found semiconscious, diaphoretic in respiratory distress by his wife twenty minutes ago. Pulsox 82 percent on room air, blood pressure 110/58, pulse around 90, respirations fluctuating from 0 to 16. IV established left forearm, 20-gauge catheter, one nitro and 80 of Lasix administered. Last BP 90/50, pulsox 96 percent with 10 liters O_2 by mask."

The medical team took over, I finished my report, Ryan took care of the truck, and Ladder 2 went back to the station.

I found out later that the patient suffered from a combination of CHF and pneumonia and his kidneys had shut down. His glucose level was 48, probably hadn't eaten in days. Cambodian people are extremely reticent about seeking Western medical care. The ER staff tried for hours to stabilize our patient. His heart stopped at around three thirty. Jess, who had taken over his care, saved him. CPR, epi, atropine, and assisted ventilations got him back again. The last I heard he was in intensive care, clinging to life with his family holding vigil.

Ouch!

We got a call for a ten-year-old boy with "pain in his genitals." What parent would call a rescue and subject their child to the humiliation of explaining his plight to more people than necessary, I wondered. We arrived at the house, a drab, three-story in a neglected neighborhood. I knocked on the door, a guy about thirty years old answered. A kitten tried to escape; the guy swatted it back in with the shirt he was holding.

The boy stood to the side, looking miserable. His mother told him to tell us what was wrong. The little guy looked down at the grimy carpet and shyly told us that his privates hurt. He noticed when he was showering. Renato, with two boys of his own back home, tried to lessen his anxiety.

"Maybe you got soap where it doesn't belong," he offered.

"I don't use soap," the kid replied, uncomfortable.

"One day I was late for work," I said as we walked outside. "I got out of the shower and was ironing my shirt naked and ironed my you-know-what by mistake."

It may have been the first time he laughed all day. I think we made a friend for life.

Seventh Floor

A world exists, parallel to our own. It is a small place, occasionally visited by people from this side. Everybody who lives there is dependent on those visits, as they are unable to care for themselves. For most, the entire life cycle begins and ends here, their time among the living brief. They are at our mercy, helpless little people who will never leave, never go to school, join a team, or win a game. They won't fall in love and get married or have a family of their own. They will never run, walk, or even learn to crawl. Some can't breathe without our help.

Children with severe disabilities live here. It is the most heartbreaking place I have ever been. The most amazing people make their living caring for them. I have no idea how they do it day after day. They become emotionally attached to every one of their patients, treating them as their own. These kids feel love every day. Twenty-four hours a day the floor is fully staffed, the need endless. Our society has evolved from survival of the fittest to where it is today, helping those unfit to survive. Are we right to prolong the lives of people who will never make it on their own? Each patient costs society millions of dollars, and the end result is always the same: they die.

At 3:00 a.m. Monday morning, I was invited to their world. One of the inhabitants, an eleven-year-old kid named

Daniel, was in respiratory distress. Renato and I rode the elevator to the seventh floor in silence, both knowing what waited on the other side of the doors. The elevator doors opened, the hissing and clicks of the respirators keeping us company as we pushed the stretcher toward our patient in the room at the end of the hall. His crib was surrounded by nurses. The respiratory therapist gave me the story. His O_2 levels had been dropping all night; all of her interventions were ineffective. He needed to be transported to Hasbro Children's Hospital.

Daniel didn't move as the therapist removed his breathing tube from the respirator and started to bag him through a stoma in his trachea. He hadn't moved on his own in eleven years. One of the nurses removed the teddy bear he had clutched to his chest. He didn't flinch. We picked him off the bed and put him on our stretcher. I noticed the pictures above his crib — birthdays, family, cards. It wouldn't be long now — different pictures on the corkboard, different family, different birthday cards, different patient.

Daniel smiled as we moved him. The nurses stroked his forehead, said they would miss him. He was aware we were moving, though he had no idea why. Back in the elevator I quickly pushed the close door button, then the ground floor, leaving his world on the seventh floor.

Gramma Muggle

Thanks to Pat Blackman, a.k.a. "Gramma Muggle," and her "Little Muggles" from Chester Barrows and Stone Hill Elementary Schools. The boxes of cards, letters, and love arrived in Iraq just in time to lift the spirits of one soldier there when he needed it most. Gramma Muggle has been a huge supporter of the Providence firefighters over the years and has extended her family to include the 1207th Transportation Company, stationed at Tallil Air Base, Iraq. People like Pat and her family make my job, and the job of everybody "over there," worth doing.

Kidnapped

We've been to the house before, ten, maybe twenty times. For thirty-eight years they lived here, bought the house when I was in the first grade. A lot of living happened here. He's in a nursing home now, the diabetes eventually taking its toll on his fragile body. He started falling, then began forgetting to take his medication. He was a US Army veteran of the Korean War.

The visiting nurses from the VA stopped coming after their patient was admitted, leaving her to fend for herself. Their middle-aged son lived on the top floor of the three-decker. He claims to be taking care of his mom, though I think the opposite is true. The lieutenant from Engine 8 gave his report as we turned onto Potters Avenue.

"Elderly lady, down on the floor for an unknown time, multiple open sores on her back, needs evaluation."

Immediately my mind flashed back to prior visits here. Her husband seemed to be the one in need of medical attention. She sat on an old, filthy chair near the front door, smiling as we worked, never saying much as we carried the man in her life past her, out the door and to the VA for treatment. I would often ask her how she was, mostly just being polite. She would smile, say "Fine," and watch us leave. Her son was always "too tired" to help or come with us as we transported his decorated war veteran dad to the hospital.

The guys from Engine 8 waited on the front porch while Lieutenant Dwyer gave us more information. I listened, but was still shocked when I saw our patient lying on her stomach in front of the filthy chair. Her urine-covered nightdress was pushed over her waist, exposing her backside and the dozens of infected sores she had been sitting on for how long, I don't know. Day, maybe week-old feces covered her feet. I took a towel from the top of her chair and, as Renato prepared to wrap her in some sheets, tried to wipe it off.

It had dried to the bottom of her feet. She screamed in pain as I wiped, skin falling off along with the mess. Renato looked at me, shook his head, and nudged me out of the way. The firefighters from Engine 8 treated her with respect and kindness as they rolled her onto her side, covered her in sheets, and placed her onto a long backboard with a cervical collar. She screamed the entire time.

"I'm not leaving!"

We kidnapped her from her own home, took her away from her son and her surroundings. I'm glad we did. She stopped screaming once we got her into the rescue, knowing her battle for independence was lost. The guys went back to the engine, a little dejected, I could tell from their somber demeanor. It can be difficult doing the right thing. We transported her to Rhode Island Hospital. I'm not sure what will become of her home, or the life she was used to.

Food

She was eighty pounds soaking wet. Quiet at first, then she opened up. She had a fever of 104 with a persistent headache. The bruises on her legs couldn't be explained. The eating disorder clinic that she was going to up until last week didn't work; she lost weight during the program. We talked about her problems. She just doesn't like to eat, she said.

I have learned a lot about eating disorders and the underlying causes that bring them on.

"The only thing you have total control over is your body and what you put into it. Sometimes that can be very comforting, but it tends to get out of control," I said as we rode toward Rhode Island Hospital. Her mouth and nose were covered with a surgical mask; her eyes grew bigger as she listened to me. I looked at her without judgment. She knew I knew.

"I lied to them at the clinic," she confessed.

"You have to tell the truth to somebody," I said.

"I did. I have a new counselor who seems to understand. I told her everything."

"You are going to feel a lot better when you can eat again," I told her, knowing not to say she would look a lot better too.

"That's what they tell me."

The health center at the college called us because they were afraid she might have meningitis. More than one health care professional told her that she is too skinny and needs to eat more. Telling somebody with an eating disorder that they are too skinny is like telling a bodybuilder he is too muscular. She needs expert help to get her back on track. I hope she finds it before she withers away.

Why We're Here
At 1800 hours we got a call for a woman in her eighties with difficulty breathing. Engine 3 got there first and gave the initial report.

"Eighty-year-old female, shortness of breath, heart rate 15 to 30."

When we entered the room I couldn't believe the woman in the bed's vitals were as bad as reported. She smiled at me and looked completely at peace. Maybe she knew something we didn't and wasn't afraid. We put her on high-flow oxygen, started an IV, and ran a 12 lead EKG. Heart rate 22, possible bundle branch block. She remained calm all the way to the trauma room.

Dr. Sullivan looked over our data and began the appropriate treatment. He told me his assessment and reasons why the patient was in the state she was in. I nodded, pretended I understood what he was saying, rubbed my chin with my thumb and index finger and said, "Of course, I agree. Thank you, Doctor."

At 1900 hours we got a call for a man unconscious on the third floor of his home. Before we arrived, Engine 10 gave us their report.

"Thirty-five-year-old male, possible OD."

Renato got the stair chair, I carried the blue bag up the stairs. The patient was in bed, diaphoretic but otherwise stable, good vitals. Renato spoke to the family and translated.

"He drank a lot."

He must have drank more than a lot. We deal with drunks all day and night; this guy was out cold, no response to verbal or painful stimuli. We carried him to the truck, worked him up and got him to the ER and into Trauma Room 2 where Dr. Sullivan took over. I again agreed with his findings.

At 2000 hours a guy called from his front porch. He was a dialysis patient having trouble breathing. Engine 10 got there first.

"Fifty-year-old male, extreme respiratory distress."

We stepped it up and found the patient doubled over on his front porch. His BP was 258/160, pulsox 82 percent. Not good. The patient was frantic, panicking. I knew Dr. Sullivan would understand. We got a driver from the 10s, kept the patient as calm as possible during the two-minute ride to the ER. This guy needed all the help he could get. My decision to "scoop and run" was what I thought would be best for the patient. We gave him a nitro and put him on O_2—no help there—and rolled. Dr. Sullivan gave him more nitro when we got there, a respiratory team was called, two IVs started, albuterol treatments, BiPAP, and more than we could have done for him. Sometimes less is more on rescue. We could have helped him breathe, but the anxiety level probably would have negated our efforts. He wanted to be in a hospital, one was two minutes away. I think we did the right thing. Dr. Sullivan seemed to agree.

2100 hours. Person unconscious, diabetic, third floor. We found a thirty-year-old guy in bed, covered in sweat and vomit, pinpoint pupils, glucose level of 20. The protocols look so easy on their nice white pages, all orderly and everything. Trying to follow them on a patient covered in vomit in an unsafe, unsanitary environment is another story. We cleaned him up the best we could, tied him onto the stair chair, and got him into the rescue, no easy task. IV, O$_2$, EKG, glucose test, vitals, 2 mg Narcan, an amp of D-50, 100 mg of thiamine and Sleeping Beauty turned into the Incredible Hulk. We held him down as best we could; security met us at the door to the ER. Dr. Sullivan looked at me and Renato when all was said and done and the patient sedated and stabilized and told us to get some rest.

Catherine

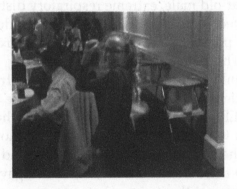

I'm sure Catherine would have preferred to have her dad escort her to Bay View's father-daughter dance but she had to put up with me instead. I know I'm a better dancer than her dad but she would never say so. Thanks, Catherine, for inviting me, and thanks to Bob and Mary for raising such a delightful young lady. Stay low, Brother, you have too much to lose.

CHAPTER 8
APRIL

Busy Day

A lot happens in the course of a day. It started at 0700, a little kid, two years old, was left in his father's car while his dad went in search of some crack cocaine. Two hours the little guy sat alone in the car until somebody called to report the situation. In a house not far away a party was going on, smoke from the marijuana covering the toddlers who lived in the house where the party went nonstop. The police were called by a concerned neighbor; they called us to have the kids taken away.

We brought them to Hasbro Children's Hospital, where they will wait for temporary foster parents to pick them up.

In a field not far away a woman, maybe a prostitute, maybe not, was being gang-raped. We were called to help an unconscious woman lying in a field. She was in her thirties, tight jeans, no shoes, ripped colorful gauze shirt. Her hair was full of dirt and leaves. She screamed "Get them off me!" all the way to the hospital. Twice she loosened the seat belts and tried to flee from the rescue as we sped through Providence. Twice I caught her just in time. The last half mile of the transport she spent on the floor at my feet, sobbing uncontrollably.

At the Providence Place Mall, a guy in his forties was getting drunk with his friends for the day until somebody snapped. Mall security called us for a man outside one of the restaurants, covered in blood. Thirty stitches should put him back together. In the West End a man was stabbed in the side. He'll probably live; we have no idea what happened. A motorcyclist lost his life on I-95 when he slammed his bike into the back of stopped traffic. Homeless people gathered at 1035 Broad Street needed to be taken to the ER three different times to sleep it off. An old lady fell, broke her hip, and was taken from her home in a stretcher, maybe the last time she will ever go through her doors.

Prisoners

He said she didn't give him his medications, she said she did. After twenty-seven years of marriage, it had come to this. For the last seven years she was his caretaker. He was confined to his bed for the most part, three heart attacks and a stroke rendering him disabled. It looked like she was running out of steam, the burden thrust upon her taking its toll. Their house was a mess — laundry, dirty dishes, paperwork, and pill bottles were strewn about haphazardly, and clutter filled the room where he spent the majority of his life. A small TV sat at the end of his bed, his portal to the world. I wonder what he watched as the days dragged on, his room more of a cell than a place to get ready for and rest from a fulfilling life.

He was hysterical, sitting up in his bed, struggling to breathe through the hole in his throat. The stoma remained clear but I was concerned that his movements would somehow clog his airway. She had a glazed look about her. At first I thought she had been drinking, because her speech was clear but slow, her pupils dilated.

"He needs to go to the hospital," she explained in a dreamy voice. "He says I didn't give him his nighttime medication, but I gave them an hour ago."

I looked on one of the dressers and saw a dozen pill bottles, some empty, others tipped on their side, duplicate prescriptions, half-eaten candy bars and trash filling every inch of the space.

"Do you have a list of his medications?" I asked. She handed me a crumbled piece of paper she picked up from the floor. Lasix, Cardizem, Zestril, Lipitor, the list was lengthy. Two names jumped off the page: Oxycontin and Vicodin. There were no bottles on the dresser that matched.

"What about these?" I asked her.

"I had to hide them. He takes thirty if I let him."

"Where are they?"

"I have them." She opened a bedroom door. A giant Rottweiler lay on the bed looking at me. She entered the room, I stayed outside as she read the names from the bottles from behind the door. She pronounced the names like she had never heard of them.

I had seen enough. We got the man ready, put him in the stair chair, and brought him out of his prison. He was crying quietly, saying he loved her and didn't want to leave his home.

I left his wife alone with her husband's prescriptions.

Air Bags

My patient was twenty-one years old, five months pregnant, and on her way to her doctor's office. She made it to the doctor's office, just not the one she had planned on. No waiting either—her condition landed her in Trauma Room 2 at Rhode Island Hospital. The air bags may have saved more than one life this day.

Jasmine

"What's your name," I asked him as we helped him down the stairs. He lost his concentration and nearly fell over as the next performer sauntered past us. Thankfully, one of us was fully focused on the job at hand and caught him before he went down. We slowly made our way down from the upper level of the club, taking in the sights when we made it to the first level. Our patient seemed unconcerned with the vomit that covered the front of his velour warm-up suit and sneakers. He had a glazed, dreamy look on his face. I asked the bouncer what happened.

"He was getting a lap dance, everything was fine, and then he stopped moving and threw up on the dancer."

"At least she won't have to wash her clothes," I mentioned as we walked under the "All Nude Room" sign at the bottom of the stairs.

"He's been drinking Heinekens and Lemon Drops," the bouncer stated as we walked into the brisk afternoon air. The fresh air did all of us some good; the perfumed atmosphere of the club had been ruined by the lemon-scented vomit on my patient. One of the dancers who had finished her shift walked past us. She did her best to attract some attention, but without the soft lighting and music the magic was gone. She became just another average-looking woman trying to make a living.

"Buddy, what's your name?" I asked again once we had him in the truck and on the stretcher. He stared at the fluorescent lights on the roof of the rig, closed his eyes, smiled and said, "Jasmine."

Broken Passport

"What's going on here?" I asked anyone who would listen. A girl of about twenty-five answered.

"My brother just found out he has AIDS. He's been crazy, he won't talk to us or let us help him."

I looked into the bedroom. Two police officers had a little man between them. They escorted him out of the destroyed room toward us. I didn't see any blood on him but you never know.

"He doesn't speak English," his sister told us as we walked him down the stairs toward the rescue. At the bottom of the stairs my patient ripped something up and threw it to the ground before getting into the truck. John, my partner for the day, went in behind him. I stopped to pick up the torn pages of his passport.

He was from Guatemala, a legal immigrant according to the document I scanned as I stepped into the truck. Thirty years old, in the country since 2005. His work boots were spattered with different color paint, his work pants worn at the knees. He sat on the bench seat and stared straight ahead. I showed him the passport I had picked up off the street. He said "Thank you," shook his head from side to side, then looked at the floor.

"It may not be as bad as you think," I offered. "They have medications now that help." He didn't understand me. I will never understand what he was feeling as I walked him into the ER, surrounded by security.

Stroke

The call was for a possible stroke at a methadone clinic. There was almost a stroke all right, but the person having it was me. We pulled the rescue to the side door of the place; we've been there numerous times and know the drill. Our patient was reported to have vomited and was feeling nausea after eating a powdered donut.

"What about the possible stroke?" I asked. The staff, nurses, psychologists, and a bunch of other educated people looked at me like I was from another planet.

"He's feeling weak," said one of them, "and not acting normally. It could be a stroke."

"It could be whooping cough," I said. We walked to the rescue. The guy was lethargic and had slurred speech. He was at least six two and weighed two twenty.

"Are you going to vomit again," I asked.

"Again?" he replied.

"Didn't you just vomit?"

"That was two days ago."

"Why are you going to the hospital?" I asked as Joe, my partner for the day, started to pull out of the parking lot.

"I'm not going anywhere!" my patient shouted. He jumped from his seat and opened the side door of the rescue. I grabbed his belt, yanked him back in, and planked him back on the seat.

"Stop the truck! Let me out! You assholes!" he shouted and tried to get up again.

"Step on it, Joe," I said. Joe stepped on the gas, the patient lost his balance and fell back onto the seat. He continued shouting. I looked at him and told him it would be in his best interests to stop acting like a baby. He stood up again and went for the door. We wrestled a little, but a heroin addict on methadone and powdered donuts is no match for a disgruntled rescue officer.

Security met us at Rhode Island Hospital and escorted our patient in. I got a coffee and waited for the next one.

Moron

These people are my friends I thought to myself as the man lying on the stretcher spit, struggled, and shouted, "Get the niggers off of me!" I stood to the side and watched as a couple of security guards applied the four-point straps that would immobilize him. "Niggers," over and over he said it. I'm sure that in the course of his normal day he would never consider saying it out loud. In his drug-crazed, drunken state, however, the word flowed freely from his mouth.

The fact that he was an idiot did nothing to lessen my unease. I considered making light of the situation later when I talked to the guards, doctors, and nurses who bore the brunt of his racist remarks but decided not to. There was nothing light about what happened.

We work together in one of the most stressful atmospheres there is. Mutual respect has been earned by the teamwork evident on a daily basis at the ER. The people here are not white, black, Hispanic, gay, or anything other than the folks I work with and trust with my life. Unfortunately, a moron comes here and reminds us we live in a world where racial divisions still exist.

It's a Boy

Well, it finally happened. A mother delivered a baby boy in the back of my rescue. I, of course, took full credit for the delivery, which was probably the single most gratifying moment of my career.

At around 7:30 last night we got a call for "a birth in progress." Engine 11 was first on scene and reported no birth; the patient was having contractions but was able to ambulate outside to the rescue. We pulled in front of the house at 7:35. The patient could make it no further than her front porch.

It is kind of strange how you just know when things have ratcheted up a notch. Al, who was working overtime, pulled the stretcher to the bottom of the six porch stairs. Miles, Drew, and Seth each grabbed an arm or a leg and helped me carry the patient Vietnam-style and drop her onto the stretcher. We had her in the truck in about a minute. Seth got the emergency OB kit ready as I did an initial assessment. I took a look and saw the baby's head.

"You're crowning," I told the mom, as if she didn't already know. She was fantastic, no screaming, all business. This was her first child. I placed my hand on the baby's head, expecting to actually do something, when out came the baby. Beautiful, pink color, I swear he opened his eyes and looked right at me.

"It's a boy," I said, my moment of glory finally upon me.

"We know," the parents said in unison, bringing me back down to earth. Al clamped the umbilical cord in the proper places and got the scalpel ready. Drew, who is expecting his first child on April 30, stopped everything.

"Let the father do it!" The father was running into the house to get his wife's glasses so she could see her son. We waited for him, only a few seconds but it seemed a lifetime, looking at a newborn still connected to his mother. The dad did his job perfectly, and Miles wrapped the newborn in a blanket and handed him up to his mom, who was absolutely radiant.

I asked permission, then took a picture with my phone. I e-mailed it to them when I got back to the station. It occurred to me later as I reflected on the whole thing that we will be a part of this family's story for a long, long time. I'm sure the story of how the baby was brought into the world in the back of a rescue will be told over and over, hopefully spanning generations. The thought of it made me realize how fortunate I am to have the greatest job in the world.

Five Years Old
A beautiful five-year-old shouldn't be unconscious at nine in the morning. She managed to get up and dressed for school but not much more. She said she was tired and went back to bed. Her mom checked on her some time later and couldn't get her up. When we got there the child was limp. We did everything we could think of, checked her glucose level, blood pressure, CO level, EKG, put her on oxygen and tried to start an IV. She didn't flinch when we put the needle in her arm.

I called Hasbro to tell them what to expect. They hear my voice so often telling them I've got a child with a fever, cough, bellyache, etc., that my report took them by surprise. "Five-year-old female, unconscious, minimal response to painful stimuli, vitals stable but otherwise unresponsive." We put the mom in back with her daughter. She was strong but shaken. I asked about seizures, medications, chemicals, anything I could think of as we transported. Nothing unusual about her history, she was fine last night.

The child went directly to the trauma room at Hasbro. There a team of doctors, nurses, respiratory people, students, and EMTs started another IV, kept the O_2 flowing, and pretty much brainstormed, trying to figure out what was going on. They took another glucose test—this time the result was 24, hypoglycemic. They administered dextrose through the IV and presto, a glorious five-year-old appeared, replacing the lifeless figure on the stretcher. She has a lot of tests to endure, but hopefully we had a happy ending.

Hmm . . .

0330. A man called from a pay phone stating he had trouble breathing. Arrived on scene at 0336. Patient stated he "smoked too many cigarettes and now couldn't breathe." What to do?

Close to Home

We do what we do so often it is easy to fall into a routine. People call 911, we respond, triage, treat, transport. The calls differ but, after years, begin to resemble one another until your shift becomes just another day at work. It is imperative we remember that there are human beings on the other end of the 911 call. What to us is another job, to the folks making the call a potentially life-changing event is unfolding.

An elderly lady in an assisted-living facility is found unresponsive on her kitchen floor. 911 is called, we respond. One look is all I need, I know this is serious. The guys from Engine 11, who just last week helped deliver a beautiful baby boy, are ready to do their thing. No words are necessary, we've been through this before. Cervical collar, backboard, oxygen, EKG, IV, contact Rhode Island Hospital en route with the information.

"Eighty-four-year-old female, unconscious, BP 184/148, normal sinus rhythm, glucose 220, pulse 84, respirations 28, ETA four minutes."

I pushed the off button on the mic and put it back in its cradle. Only then did I see the name on the report. My sister Melanie's mother-in-law. I think my heart hit the floor of the rescue. I looked at my patient's face. Peaceful and serene, though her body was experiencing life-threatening damage. The guys from Engine 11 and Mark from Rescue 1, B group, did their thing (Renato had a crisis of his own, our prayers are with his family), switching oxygen bottles, monitoring the vitals, and getting ready to transfer our patient from the rescue to the hospital. I watched from the captain's chair and thought of the times I was in Hannah's company. I smiled when I remembered her unfaltering faith in God. Whatever the outcome, she is in good hands.

I called Mel from the trauma room and told her the bad news. Good luck, Bob, Mel, and the Frasier family. Our thoughts are with you during this difficult time.

Vindicated

For two days he endured the pain. Every time he tried to pee he was reminded that everything wasn't "okay." Finally, he called his son and daughter to his apartment on the second floor and told them the truth. They tried to help him down the stairs into their car but he couldn't make it. Time had ravaged his once powerful body, that and a debilitating stroke he had while at the hardware store on Valentine's Day. Now he sat in bed, unable to pee or do much of anything for that matter.

He lost his wife two years ago, then his daughter last year. Old age took the love of his life, and breast cancer took one of the ten products of that love. The others, seven girls and two boys, were also born during their marriage, one that spanned six decades. The pictures that covered the apartment showed a beautiful life together.

His youngest daughter who rode in the back of the rescue and told me their story thought her dad was dying of a broken heart. Since he lost his wife and daughter, all he did was cry. Now, he thought he had prostate cancer. In a way, he was relieved; some men prefer to bear the pain for their family rather than see them suffer. Maybe he felt vindicated now that he felt his loved ones' pain, in his mind forgiven for failing them.

CHAPTER 9
MAY

Different Worlds
At 0330 hours, Rescue 1 responded to a home on Blackstone Boulevard for a fifty-two-year-old female suffering from back pain. We arrived at 0335. The groundskeeper met us at the end of the driveway and escorted us past a Bentley and a Mercedes, through a beautifully landscaped entryway, and to an ornate fifteen-foot door. Once inside the foyer, a grand staircase adorned with valuable works of art led us to our patient. She was a pleasant woman, lying on her back in the hallway grimacing in pain. It appeared she slipped a disc. Her dog, a purebred, perfectly manicured non-shedding poodle-thing, stayed by her side but didn't threaten. We put the lady on a backboard and carried her through her million-dollar house and into the rescue. She was a good sport, enduring our teasing as we transported her to Miriam Hospital for treatment.

An hour later we received another call, less than a mile away. The three-decker was dark, the stairs creaky. A man in his fifties sat at a lonely kitchen table waiting for us to check his blood sugar. He had been feeling weak and worried he might pass out and nobody would find him. He lived alone, his apartment smaller than the entryway of our last patient's home. The man was a gracious host; he seemed to enjoy the company. He lives a solitary life here on the outskirts of the opulent East Side mansions in a modest home on what I'm sure is a small fixed income. His glucose level was within normal range. He wished us good-night and locked the door behind us.

Two patients, two different worlds less than a mile apart. They both seemed happy in their place, neither concerned with, or even aware of, the other world that exists right outside their doorway.

Eye Opener

He was keeled over a fallen utility pole, his ass in the air and his face on the ground. His associates were putting the finishing touches on a half-gallon jug of vodka.

"He's drunk," said one of them as we stood there mustering the energy to take him away. It was seven thirty; we had been going nonstop for twenty-four and a half hours. The first of the month coupled with a full moon puts money in the pockets of crazy people.

"No shit," I said, then grabbed the guy's belt and dumped him onto the stretcher. Their sunrise party continued while we wheeled our patient off the field. The half gallon was almost empty; the remaining two might make it until noon before they passed out.

Mark got the guy's vital signs while I filled out the report. Things were mostly normal; the only potential problem was his glucose level, 58. He slept peacefully while we transported him to Rhode Island Hospital.

We rolled him through the doors of the ER and transferred him to a hospital stretcher. While I gave my report, one of his eyes popped open.

"Fifty-four-year-old male found sleeping in a field, no sign of trauma, history of alcohol abuse, admits to drinking, vitals stable but his blood sugar is a little low."

The drunk guy opened his other eye and said in a gravelly voice, "My sugar's low and my alcohol is high!" He then laughed himself into unconsciousness. They put some orange juice on his stretcher and put him in with the rest of them.

Must the Show Go On?
I really don't know what to make of this. We got a call this morning for a man down. Get there and find a fifty-five-year-old guy dead in bed. The family was hysterical, nothing we could do. The guy's wife looked familiar; I found out later that she works in one of the area emergency rooms. Their son's wedding is supposed to be today, family from out of town was at the house, the flowers, band, reception, limos, cake, and everything else was waiting. The guy had no significant history, just partied the night before at the rehearsal dinner. If I was the guy who died, I'd want the show to go on. What do you think?

Raid
Somebody at 177 Julian called 911, that much we know. When the guys from Ladder 6 arrived, nobody answered the door. They did what any self-respecting ladder company would do—they proceeded to force their way into the house. One of the guys went for a window while the others worked on the back door. They popped it open, right into the forehead of the little old lady who was hiding behind it. She yelled for a while but nobody could understand her. Eventually her daughter came along and explained things.

A few months ago the house was raided by the police. They had the wrong information and were looking for drugs that weren't there. The poor lady thought we were the cops coming to raid the place again. It's a good thing she wasn't armed or a real tragedy could have occurred. Eventually things got back to normal. The guys from Atwells Avenue went back to their station to finish their lunch, although I heard later that the Explorers, six teenaged kids who had visited the station, ate every crumb. No rescue was needed, the lady and her daughter went back inside, hopefully with no hard feelings. We never did find out who called us, another unsolved mystery in a city full of them.

Retired

"Rescue 1 and Engine 13, respond to Homer Avenue for a diabetic."

5:30 a.m. Cinco de Mayo was thankfully over for this year. Thirty-four runs in thirty-eight hours, most alcohol related. This should be our last call, then three days off. Engine 13 was first on scene.

"Engine 13 to fire alarm, advise rescue we have a fifty-seven-year-old male, confined to bed with a blood glucose of 12."

Great.

"Rescue 1, received, on scene."

My partner for the night, Steve Whalen, usually assigned to Engine 13 but detailed to Rescue 1 for the night because of lack of manpower, got the stair chair from the back compartment and I grabbed the blue bag.

"I've been here before," said Steve as we made our way into the house.

A hospital bed was set up in the living room, a bag of food attached to a pole stood nearby. The patient, a young-looking fifty-seven-year-old, was diaphoretic and unconscious. I decided to treat him immediately. We started an IV after a few misses and got the D-50 ready. The man's family stood by silently as we worked. Steve had the medication ready, I pushed the contents of the vial through the IV line and into the patient's bloodstream.

"When was the last time anybody saw him awake?" I asked.

"Last night," said his wife.

Her husband's eyes started blinking, then stayed open. He stared into space for a few minutes before regaining consciousness.

"Has he been eating properly?" I asked. His wife pointed to the feeding tube. Enough said.

"What hospital does he go to?" I asked.

"I don't want him to go to the hospital. We can take care of him here."

"He should go," I argued. "He needs to have blood work done, maybe his medications need tweaking."

"Please, let him stay," said the man's wife. I got the refusal form ready for her to sign. "No transport against medical advice."

The family thanked us, greatly appreciative of the job we did. Their father, husband, and friend was conscious again, drinking a glass of juice. On the way back to the station, Steve told me the rest of the story.

"He fell down his cellar stairs about two months ago," he said. "Nobody knew it but he was there for hours. He had a major head bleed. He was going to retire this year after twenty-five years working at the prison. He's paralyzed, probably for life."

I forgot how tired I was as I walked up the stairs back to my office, thankful just to be able to make the steps. I have a bad habit of looking toward the finish line instead of enjoying the ride. Retirement will come soon enough. I hope it's worth working for.

Note to Self . . .
When you spot a building fire while driving down Route 10, figure out where, or even kind of where, said fire is located before getting on the radio and letting the entire shift know you have no idea whatsoever where you are going.

The fire was in Olneyville. The guys from Atwells Avenue, Engine 14 and Ladder 6, saw the smoke from their station and got there right before we did. They had it under control in less than a half hour, a pretty good job considering the house was nearly fully involved when I saw it from the highway.

Benjamin

Our patient lived above a restaurant on Wickenden Street, one of the more "hip" spots in Providence. Traffic was tight, the sidewalk busy while people shopped and relaxed at the many coffee shops, art galleries, and antique stores that line the street. We had to block the travel lane when we stopped the rescue at our destination.

As soon as we stopped, three Japanese sushi chefs escorted an older guy from their doorway. He was limping; our patient. He owned the building and rented the lower floor to a popular Japanese restaurant. From the concern showed by his tenants he was a well-liked landlord. I knew right away I was going to enjoy this call—the guy had character written all over his craggy face. He hobbled up the rescue steps, no easy task for somebody half his age with two good wheels, and sat on the stretcher.

"What's the matter?" I asked him.

"My leg is swollen and my toe hurts. It's been going on for weeks. I'm leaving for Europe tomorrow, I hope I can make the trip."

I took a look at the leg and toe. His left calf and shin were twice the size of the right and his big toe was bright red.

"How are you going to get around Europe on that?" I asked.

"Don't know. Can you take me to the VA?"

We took his vital signs and got going. Ben was a Navy man, WWII vet, disabled. He was there at Normandy on D-Day, lost some friends as wave after wave debarked from his ship into the slaughterhouse. When that job was done he went to the Pacific and was training to parachute onto Japan when the bomb was dropped and the war ended. He spent a lot of the war with the Merchant Marines, a group who suffered staggering losses during the war. He survived the war; sadly, his brother did not. Ben told me about him.

"He was a gifted musician and brilliant Brown grad whose life was cut short in the Black Forest during the Battle of the Bulge." I thought of my own brother, fighting the war in Iraq and the loss my family would suffer if he doesn't make it home. All of these years have passed yet Ben's eyes still filled up when he mentioned his brother.

"My father is a Navy vet, Korea, and my brother is in Iraq," I mentioned, proud of my family's accomplishments. We talked a little more during the trip to the VA. Thankfully for us, Ben lived through the war. He taught art at the Rhode Island School of Design, displayed his work at galleries throughout Providence, and is a successful restaurateur.

I can only imagine what contributions to society have been lost, greatness unknown, and words unspoken. How much more music will we never hear, art we will never see, or lives we won't be able to share and enjoy before the world makes peace with itself?

God, I hate this war. Five soldiers dead, three missing this morning west of Baghdad.

Ball Three

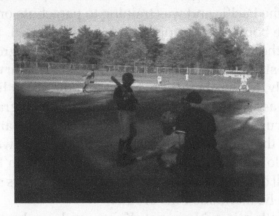

Nothing better on a beautiful spring night than a ball game! It would have been better if Renato's oldest son's team didn't get whooped. Doesn't matter, though. We enjoyed an inning and a half before a call came to take us back to reality.

John

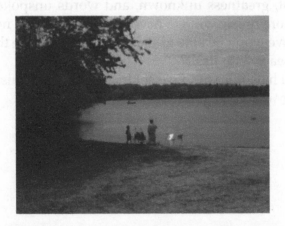

As I walked Zimba and Lakota along the shore of Gorton Pond, I came across these two, a father and son feeding the swans. Jeff, my friend and sometime partner on Rescue 1, spends a lot of time with his newborn son, John. He was born prematurely right around the time me and Al delivered another baby inside the rescue. He now lives in a controlled environment at Women and Infants Hospital.

I'm sure Jeff and Maria long for the day when they can take their baby home, hold him and see his face unencumbered by breathing devices. It must be torture for them to watch their child grow, close to them yet still distant in the hospital's sterile atmosphere. Jeff's holding up well, though unfortunately for him he had to learn the frustration and pain of fatherhood before experiencing the joy. That joy is coming, buddy, and it is well worth the wait.

Crackhead

He was handcuffed, sitting in the back of a police cruiser on a rainy Wednesday night. His eyes rolled back in his head and drool ran off his chin onto a white T-shirt that said in bold black letters, "Grow Up."

"What happened to him?" I asked one of the cops.

"He might have swallowed a rock."

"How long ago?"

"No more than ten minutes."

I reached in and helped our newfound patient to his feet. He stumbled into the rescue, claimed he had chest pain, blurred vision, difficulty breathing, and a migraine headache. He started to thrash around the stretcher, moaning and drooling some more. When his convulsions stopped we took some vital signs. BP 148/98, heart rate of 120, glucose 104, SpO_2 98 percent.

"What's wrong with him?" somebody asked.

"Crackhead."

When we were done our patient went catatonic. Better for me—it kept him quiet during transport to Rhode Island Hospital.

Graduation!
Friday, May 18, 2007.

Happy ending!

I received a phone call and thank-you card from Kellie's family yesterday. It is my pleasure to tell you that she will graduate from Providence College this Sunday. Despite the hardships she endured and long road to recovery, she made the dean's list. Congratulations, Kellie!

Not many are able to recover from bacterial meningitis, let alone finish school. The students at North Providence High School where Kellie interned had no idea of the difficult road their new mentor traveled to get to them. They and her future students will benefit from the wisdom and strength only one who fought and won such a courageous battle can pass on.

Thank you, Patti Coughlin and family. Their thoughtfulness is greatly appreciated. I passed on the well-wishes to the guys who were there with us on that Tuesday in September. It is great to know that the Providence Fire Department is held in such high regard by the Coughlins. With all the terrible things we see daily, their story reminds us that we do make a difference, and people appreciate us. In their own way, they helped us as much as we helped them.

Twilight Zone
He showed up with his new girlfriend at his son's mother's house to take her to work. His son's mother said something about the girlfriend. They fought in the stairway of the apartment. The son's mother's sister woke up, heard the fighting, and tried to stop it. The father choked both women and smashed the sister's head into the doorjamb, causing a

three-inch laceration that would require stitches. The son's mother ran downstairs and called 911.

By the time we got there, the cops had both parents in cuffs in back of separate cruisers. The present girlfriend still sat in the father's car in front of the baby's mother's house. The girlfriend in the car needed to get home to babysit for her son's father's other son. Two beautiful boys, three and four years old, watched all of this, one walking around the apartment with a confused look on his face, the other being held by one of the cops, a monster of a man who nobody in their right mind would antagonize. I thought Rod Serling from *The Twilight Zone* was going to materialize from thin air and say, "You unlock this door with the key of imagination. Beyond it is another dimension . . ."

Renato got the baby's mother into the rescue and cleaned her head laceration. I made arrangements with the police to drop the boys off at their grandmother's house on the way to the emergency room. Once inside the safety of the rescue, I found that the twenty-one-year-old mother was a pleasant young lady whose only worry was that she wasn't going to be able to shop for her son's birthday party this Saturday. She wanted him to know that he was special on his special day. She worked part time at Burger King, and part time at the local youth center as a lifeguard.

I wish *The Twilight Zone* door would open and take these people away from here, into a place where they have a chance. This neighborhood is going to swallow them whole and spit out the broken pieces. It's only a matter of time.

Wake Up!
They came from Coventry, a suburb of Providence, looking for some heroin. They found it, more than they bargained for it turns out. Witnesses saw a car stop in a parking lot, dump a guy out one of the back doors, then speed away. The guy

dumped in the parking lot wasn't breathing. Friends like these . . .

Engine 10 was first on scene responding from the Broad Street station, less than a mile away. Rescue 1 is located about five minutes away, and we were speeding toward the scene when Captain Cunha radioed the message.

"Twenty-year-old male, respiratory arrest, possible OD."

"Rescue 1, received." I put the mic back into the cradle and let Renato drive. Two minutes later we arrived on scene. The guys from Engine 10 had established a line and pushed 2 mg of Narcan into the vein of the unconscious kid. A minute later he started breathing on his own. A minute after that he opened his eyes and looked around, no idea what had happened or how close to death he was. Had his "friends" dumped him in a field or deserted street he would not have lived to tell the tale to his "friends" back in Coventry.

We transported him to Rhode Island Hospital. When the Narcan wears off, sometimes the patient goes back into respiratory arrest. At first he was polite and thankful; by the time we got him to the hospital he was back to normal, asking how long he was going to be stuck at the hospital. He wanted to get back to Coventry.

If he comes back to Providence, I hope he doesn't end up in a body bag.

Meeting

Meeting somebody who has made a huge emotional impact on you is difficult enough; doing so in front of news cameras is altogether different! I met Kellie and her family on Saturday. Channel 12 News did a story about her, describing her ordeal and miraculous recovery. It was a good story, and I'm glad I took part in the production. Had I not, I never would have met the Coughlins. It was a meeting I will never forget, one of the highlights of my career. We all survived the TV ordeal, and when it was over Kellie and her clan went to dinner at one of Providence's best restaurants. I got back in the rescue and headed toward home, feeling better than I had in a long time. I may never see them again, but now that our paths have crossed I think we are all better because of it.

Grounded

"Rescue 1 to fire alarm, are the police on the way?"

"They've been notified."

"I've got an angry, intoxicated man with a big rock giving me a hairy eyeball."

"The police are on the way."

"Can you have them step it up? Disregard, I have a visual."

I rolled the window down a crack and yelled at the man holding the rock:

"Put down the rock!"

He sneered at me and reared his arm back. I rolled the window back up and waited for the glass to shatter. When it didn't, I rolled the window back down a crack and repeated:

"Put down the rock!"

The maniac saw the cops coming, threw the rock to the curb, and started to walk away. The officer grabbed him and brought him back to us.

"Did he threaten you guys?" the cop asked while frisking his prisoner, smashing a crack pipe on the street, then dumping the guy's lighter. No rocks, he must have smoked it all.

Before I could answer, a friend of the rock-throwing, crack-smoking, vodka-guzzling nut showed up.

"I'll take him home, he's just messed up," said the man's friend. Suddenly he looked like a sad old man, beaten and dejected. He was out of crack, out of money, no more booze, and about to be arrested.

"Nah, I don't think he even knows what he's doing," I told the police.

The cop let him go, making the man's friend promise to take him home and keep him there.

Hearing Voices

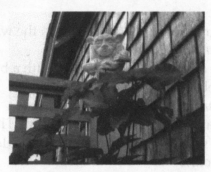

I was leaving for work at sunrise, Saturday, Memorial Day weekend, seventy degrees, low humidity, not a cloud in the sky. A little voice told me it might be better to stay home.

Deserved Rest

Welcome home, Bob! It took three days to get from Iraq to Rhode Island. Fifteen days leave during a five hundred–day deployment in a war zone doesn't seem like much but I'm sure he'll take it. Three months to go when he gets back. Maybe the war will be over by then.

Doubt it. It looks like this is going to go on for a long, long time. Eleven more soldiers killed this week, no idea how many injured. It's easy to forget that for some the war is more than news reports or fodder for political debate. Thanks again to everybody making the sacrifice and making us proud.

I'm hoping to get a round of golf in with Bob. We'll see if Mary and the kids let him out of their sight for long enough.

Captain Vernon's House

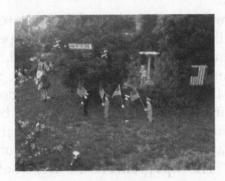

We were staged at Public and Prairie waiting for the police to secure the scene of a suicidal person when I noticed this. Turns out the property is owned by retired Providence Fire Department captain Ray Vernon's mother and sister.

No suicide, just somebody looking for attention.

Father of the Year

The guy drove an $80,000 Mercedes. Apparently, his two-year-old daughter wasn't worth the fifty bucks he would have had to spend on a car seat. She was injured by the side-impact air bags that deployed when the car collided in an intersection with a van. The beautiful little girl had only a scrape on her shoulder, but it could have been a lot worse.

A two-year-old in a speeding, unregistered, uninsured Mercedes driven by a guy with no license without a car seat.

Her father talked nonstop on his cell phone in the back of the rescue while we cared for his daughter. She was a real charmer, smiled the whole time while her dad talked to whoever about the money he was going to make from the "stupid bitch" that hit him. He wanted to know if we could stop by his daughter's mother's place of work so she could go to the hospital with the girl and he could "take care of some business."

I couldn't wait to get him out of the truck so I complied; it was only a little out of the way. Cindy stopped the rescue at a hair salon where the girl's mom worked. She got into the back accompanied by another beautiful girl, this one almost four. Dad got out, I slammed the door shut. He was about thirty years old, smart enough to be driving an $80,000 car but not bright enough to register it or insure it. His license was suspended also, but he was going to "make some money." The cops promised me they would meet us at Hasbro Children's Hospital and make an arrest. I hope they follow through.

"The problem with the human gene pool is there is no lifeguard." Whoever came up with that one got it right.

Visit

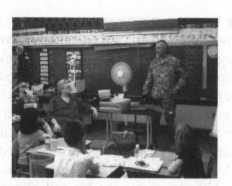

Yesterday the once notorious, feared, and downright incorrigible "Morse Brothers" visited Chester Barrows School in Cranston as guests of "Gramma Muggle," a.k.a. Pat Blackman, friend and fierce supporter of our troops and the Providence Fire Department.

Her "Little Muggles" have been sending letters and treats to the soldiers in the 1207th for a while now, much appreciated I'm told. My brother, Bob, did a great job entertaining the kids and answering an endless torrent of questions. He presented the school with a certificate of appreciation from his unit, signed by the big shots, as well as a Muslim prayer rug embroidered with thanks from the 1207th in English and Arabic. Unfortunately, a visit to Stone Hill School wasn't possible due to time restraints, but Bob presented Gramma Muggle with a certificate and prayer rug for them as well.

As I sat off to the side, I was happy to let Bob have the spotlight. He and his fellow soldiers have earned all the praise and respect that comes their way. It was a good day for us and the kids as well. I think that seeing the person they wrote their letters to gave the kids a better understanding of the sacrifices being made by folks a lot like their own parents, siblings, aunts, and uncles.

CHAPTER 10
JUNE

Atlas Shrugged

Just wondering: How did a nice old lady have a CVA on May 5 in the Dominican Republic, get on a flight to the US of A, get from the airport to her family's house, but then need to call 911 for a two-mile ride to the emergency room? I asked her family what prompted the emergency; they said she has weakness on her right side. When asked if this was a new development, they gave me a blank stare and said, "She had a stroke on May 5," as if that explained everything.

Our health care system is in shambles in large part because of these situations. Unable to get quality medical care, including physical and speech therapy, in the Dominican Republic, the family arranged for the non-English-speaking lady to come here, be transported by an emergency vehicle to an emergency room, and be entitled not only to immediate care but all the subsequent follow-up care. All this having never stepped foot in the country until yesterday. I wonder how long we can bear the weight of the world before we collapse.

Gone

Strange how chilly the night had become. A few hours ago the warm night air was full of heat and humidity. I closed the passenger-side window as we sped toward the house where a young woman was reported to be having a seizure. John McGovern was behind the wheel, both of us working our seventeenth hour of a twenty-four.

"I've been here before," he said as we stopped in front of a little one-family house on a quiet street in the city's Mount Pleasant section.

"Yup, this is the house," he mumbled to himself. We walked past the trash that had been placed at the curb for pick-up. I noticed what looked like a brand new crib, taken apart, the sides and mattress leaning against a ruined couch, the fabric of the couch ripped, it's stuffing torn out. I didn't think the crib would be here long, somebody would snatch it.

Lieutenant Rondeau walked out of the house and gave me an update on the patient's condition. It didn't appear to be a seizure, he said. I entered the house; a twenty-two-year-old woman lay on a different couch, her aunt kneeling before her, holding her hand.

"She's all right," said the aunt. "Sorry to bother you, I thought she wasn't breathing."

We did an evaluation, decided that there was no emergency, and walked out of the house past the discarded crib toward the rescue. John was unusually quiet as we rode back to the station. Halfway there, he told me the story.

"Last week we were there, her baby died on her chest while she was sleeping," he said in a low voice. I didn't interrupt, letting him tell the story at his own pace. "I think that was the couch at the curb, all slashed up, and the crib must be the baby's. We did CPR and got her to Hasbro but it was too late. I think the baby had been gone for a while." He drove slowly toward home. "Chris ran out of the house holding the baby, doing compressions. I bagged her all the way to the hospital, there was nothing we could do," he said. I wondered if he believed that or was coping the best he could. He's got a couple kids of his own.

"Did you see the crib? And the couch? That was strange," he said, shaking his head.

I agreed. He backed the rescue into the bay and headed upstairs.

Eye Infection

"Eye infection? Her eyes had better be falling out of their sockets, calling 911 at three thirty in the morning for an eye infection. Eye infection . . . Who in their right mind would call 911 at three thirty in the morning for an eye infection? I'll give her an eye infection. She'll wish she didn't have eyes when I get there. Eye infection. Unbelievable!"

"Are you done yet?" asked John as he drove toward the house. He was as tired as I was, only handling it better. It had been a grueling shift; this was our tenth run since five, our third since midnight. We had both worked all day as well.

"Almost. I know," I said, doing my best crazy lady imitation, "I'll call 911 because I have an eye infection!"

We pulled up to a dark house on a dark street. I saw a handwritten sign taped to the side of the door under a couple of doorbells that said "Apartment 2." I rang the bell closest to the sign, then read the rest of the note.

"Over There!" with an arrow pointing to the next door. Oops. Apparently we weren't the only late-night visitors here.

We stood in front of apartment 2. I rang the bell. A middle-aged lady answered, dressed in flannel pajamas, smoking a cigarette, and holding a crate of medications. She had oozing sores all over her face.

"What happened to your face?" I asked.

"I pick my skin, it got all infected. I picked this one," she pulled back a bloody scab over her left eye, "the pus ran into my eye."

Just when I thought I had seen everything.

How About a Salad

I was working with Jeff the other night and spent a lot of our shift looking for Kevin. You may remember him from previous posts—he's the guy that drinks himself into unconsciousness, then pops up when we least expect it and asks trivia questions. "Whose the guy . . ."

Jeff had a bag of clothes to give him. We do a lot of complaining about the drunks and abuse of the 911 system, but some of us actually care about the welfare of our most annoying patients. They truly cannot take care of themselves. What promise they once had has been drowned by years of alcohol abuse. Is there redemption? I honestly hope so.

Al and Jeff, partners on Rescue 1, D group, have not given up hope. Neither is timid when it comes to expressing an opinion or dealing with combative patients, but there is a side to them that shows through their rough exterior whether they like to let it out or not. I've noticed that most Providence firefighters are like that—when you least expect it, at times from the least likely person, an act of kindness will appear that reaffirms my faith in the goodness of humanity. This is just the most recent example.

One of our regular drunks was passed out in the Wendy's parking lot. Somebody called 911, Al and Jeff responded. The guy was only a "little" intoxicated, probably enough to knock most of us senseless. He asked Jeff for some money. "Why don't I buy you a burger instead," Jeff said. "That way you won't buy another bottle of vodka." The drunk thought about it for a minute and said, "No thanks. There's a lot of saturated fat in hamburg, and it's not real meat. Who knows what kind of chemicals are in those things."

"Well what do you want?" Jeff asked.

"How about a salad?"

They got the drunk his salad and went back in service.

Beats War

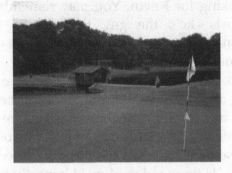

A bad day golfing is better than a good day at war. I hope Bob's better with his weapons than he is with his golf clubs. We pretty much stunk up the Exeter Country Club but had a ball doing it.

Missed Chance

We sat next to each other on the curb in front of his grandfather's house. He was about ten years old, barely holding back a flood of tears. His sister wasn't able to control her emotions, her tears flowed freely.

"He was fine last night," she said. "How could he die?"

We got the call at 0658 for a man not breathing. Engine 13 led the way down the tree-lined street near the Cranston line; we followed a safe distance behind. In the distance, past the engine I saw frantic motion in front of a nice two-story Cape. As we approached I saw the kids waving us in.

The boy had gone to wake his grandfather as he does every day for a ride to school.

"I knew something was wrong when I saw his eyes open and not blinking," he said between sobs. "He goes to work every day. He can't be gone."

He sat next to me for a while, rocking gently, side to side. He pulled his knees toward his chest and hugged them. All I wanted to do was put my arm around his shoulders, give him some comfort, maybe make his pain more bearable. Instead I looked toward Broad Street for the police sergeant to come and take over. I wish I had taken the chance. I don't know if I was afraid of scaring him, or hurting myself if he were to stiffen and walk away. An uncomfortable silence lasted for about a minute. Then he got up and walked into the house. A few minutes later, his sister followed.

The police arrived at 0715. I told them the time of death and went home. Days later I still feel as though I failed. I had a chance to help those kids but for whatever reason chose not to. I'm sure there will be more death and heartache to deal with. Maybe next time I won't be as afraid.

Drowning

For nine years I have walked through these sliding glass doors. Nothing much had changed in the three years since I had last entered here. The first floor was still empty. The elevators still painfully slow.

A lady on the fourth floor was in congestive heart failure. I had received her vital signs over the radio from Elliot, the lieutenant from Engine 12. Not good: blood pressure 212/120, pulsox 79 percent, rapid heart rate. Her lungs were filling with fluid, making each breath she took harder and harder. I've heard that it feels like drowning to the person experiencing the symptoms. The fourth floor is where patients suffering from dementia and Alzheimer's disease live. I imagine the patient had no idea what was going on; she could think she was drowning in the ocean for all we knew.

Finally the elevator stopped on the first floor. Me and Vicro, my new partner — Renato has flown the coup (that's another story)—rolled the stretcher in and hit the up button. The doors opened on the fourth floor, home for the twenty or so residents here. The place is immaculate, floors shined, flowers in vases here and there, and a birdcage on a table in the foyer. The birds were sleeping. So were most people. It was two thirty in the morning.

I entered the room. The patient lay in her bed, an unknowing look of worry on her face. The guys from Engine 12 had her on oxygen and ready to be transferred to my stretcher. Her name was Eileen. I told her what was happening as we moved her over. Even though she was drowning in her own fluid, I think she relaxed a little, knowing we were there to help. We packed up our stuff, med bags, defibrillator, and oxygen tank and headed for the elevator. The nurse on the floor followed us down the corridor.

"Bye, Eileen, see you when you get back," she said, insincerity evident in her tone. She looked me in the eye and said conspiratorially, "If you get back," and smiled.

My mother spent her last nine years of her life here, dying in one of these rooms the week before Christmas. I'm not proud to say I imagined the nurse on the stretcher, full of tubes and drowning in her own sarcasm.

We got Eileen to the hospital after treating her in front of the nursing home for about fifteen minutes. Vicro established an IV, we gave her nitro, aspirin, 40 mg of Lasix, and an albuterol treatment. Her pulsox was 93 percent with a blood pressure of 170/100 when we left.

She'll be back.

Moment of Silence

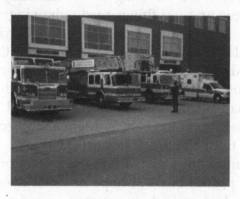

May the spirit of the nine firefighters from Charleston, South Carolina, live on forever . . .

Washington Street, moment of silence in honor of the deceased, 19 June 07, 1900 hours.

Peanuts

Traffic was slow, a combination of construction projects, a few accidents, and the lethargy that a beautiful day brings on. We needed to get from South Providence over to Mount Pleasant, a trip of about ten miles, as quickly as possible. An eleven-month-old infant was waiting. The report said he was having trouble breathing and had hives on his face, chest, and back. Vicro hit the gas, forcing cars out of our way with the lights and sirens, clearing a path as best he could. An infant having an allergic reaction is potentially fatal, and there was no way a baby was going to die on my watch. All of our rescues were tied up on other calls and two or three out-of-town rescues were covering the runs that we couldn't get to. Though it was on the opposite end of the city, this one was ours.

Joe from Engine 6 gave me an update when we arrived in front of the house, telling me the baby's face was swelling and the hives were traveling down his body. I climbed into the rescue and got things ready, drawing up .1 mg of epinephrine, 1/1000 into a 3 ml syringe, hooked a pediatric nasal cannula up to the O$_2$ port, and prepared the stretcher. Vicro carried the baby into the truck, the mother and sister followed. Hives had appeared all over his body and slight wheezing had begun. I told the mom what I was doing, prepared the site on the baby's thigh, and injected the epi. Vicro got in front and drove toward Hasbro.

Peanut butter crackers were the culprit. Aton had never before tried peanut butter. I hope he never does again. His eyes, which had puffed up, started to return to normal and the redness and swelling on his face diminished. The wheezing disappeared as well. The mom was relieved, the sister too, but most of all the guy in charge of the rescue. We took him to Hasbro for an evaluation and got ready for the next call.

Choking

I've got an eleven-month-old infant properly restrained in the captain's seat, looking at me, an earring lodged in her throat, a hysterical mother insisting on holding her baby in her arms during transport, a ten-minute ride to Hasbro Children's Hospital. Every now and then the baby holds her breath and looks shocked, then breathes again. John, my driver, is doing his best to beat the rush hour traffic on Route 10. A moron refuses to yield the right of way, pulls next to the rescue and flips off John, still refuses to get out of the way. Meanwhile I'm on the phone with the doctor from Hasbro explaining that my patient has a partially obstructed airway, a sharp object lodged in her throat, and occasional difficulty breathing. The mother is screaming at me to do something, telling John to go faster, while the doctor wants to know the child's vital signs, like I have time for that. I'm preparing the ET kit just in case even though I've never intubated a child, the moron is now following us and making a real ass of himself, the baby's face turns red, her eyes tear up, she coughs, then closes her eyes and doesn't make a sound. I feel the truck turn, then feel the familiar bumps of the highway off ramp and know the hospital is seconds away. The baby burps, smiles, and starts to breathe normally. The truck backs into the bay at Hasbro.

A day later I get a call from the EMS chief wanting an explanation concerning our behavior against a citizen who filed a formal complaint against us for harassing him on the highway. The whole incident will be dropped if we just "tell the truth."

I GOT YOUR TRUTH, RIGHT HERE!

Summer Fun

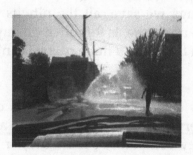

Trooper

A Rhode Island state trooper has spent the last ten days at Rhode Island Hospital recovering from a life-threatening blow to the face and subsequent fall to the back of his head. Our guys responded, did their job, IV, O$_2$, EKG, immobilization, and transport, in incredible time. The doctors at the ER credited Rescue 4 and Engine 3 with saving the trooper's life.

His pupils were blown, blood pouring from the ears, nose, and mouth, when we arrived. He was given last rites and organ donation was being considered. Luckily our rescue was available on a Saturday night at closing time. We scooped him up and, with help from the firefighters on Engine 3, did our thing while en route to the trauma room, five minutes away.

The trooper is twenty-five and in great shape, which helps. The state cops I run into can't thank us enough. The trooper's family treats us like miracle workers. It is very humbling, but greatly appreciated.

Today I visited the intensive care unit with the guy in charge of the rescue that night. The trooper's mother, father, and brother were there and we talked for a while. He is going to be extubated tomorrow, is responding to questions by squeezing hands, and opens his eyes. They are hopeful for a full recovery. Extensive therapy is in his future but it looks like he is going to make it.

All the assbags we save, all the nitwits we take to the hospital, all the nonsense, is forgotten on days like this. The family plans on throwing a huge party. I can't wait.

Cashed Out

The firefighters did their job, the patients chose to ignore their advice. Cervical collars are applied to any victim of an MVA when they complain of neck and/or back pain. The driver and front seat passenger of a car that was struck while stopped at a stop sign said they were hurt, and they were treated accordingly.

When Rescue 1 arrived, about ten minutes after Engine 12, the "injured" were walking around the scene. One of them actually went into a local convenience store to buy some cigarettes, both wearing the bulky white collars that are designed to keep the neck immobilized and prevent further spinal cord damage. We rounded them up, put them on spine boards, immobilized them the rest of the way, and headed out toward Rhode Island Hospital.

The female victim talked on the phone for a bit while I gathered her friend's information. She was excited, talked about the big payday when she sued the morons who crashed into her. She could barely contain herself she was so happy. Her friend was a little more subdued, just answered my questions. We rode toward the hospital, me writing the facts of the accident on the state report, them talking about who they were going to sue.

As we approached the ramp to the ER her phone rang one more time. They were towing her car! She was furious! How dare they! The car wasn't insured or registered but hey, that's not their problem. Some idiot hit them! Can you believe this bullshit!

I couldn't stop laughing as we carried them in.

CHAPTER 11
JULY

Look What I Found

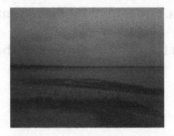

Back to work tomorrow. I finally found time to take the dogs for a walk . . . look what I found! I knew the water was around here somewhere, just didn't know the serenity and view would be so nice. The picture was taken from Gaspee Point. In the distance is East Providence, with a little of Providence on the left. The dogs went fishing; I just took it all in.

A quick twenty-four-hour shift tomorrow, a few days off, then back to the grind until fall. The move went well, all things considered. Feels like a fresh start.

Home Sweet Home

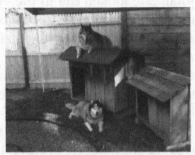

Zimba and Lakota have settled in nicely. Cheryl and Michael still have a way to go!

Troubled

She was handcuffed, lying facedown on the floor, surrounded by cops, firefighters, and social workers.

"Watch her, she spits," said one of her counselors when I helped her to her feet.

"She needs a psych eval," said another counselor, handing me a package of paperwork.

I took a quick look at the information and found what I was looking for.

"Danielle, what's going on here?" I asked, keeping my distance.

"These assholes don't listen! Big tough guys beating up a little girl!" She glared at the police.

I glanced back at the paperwork and saw her medications. Depakote, Clonipin, Prozac, lithium, birth control.

We walked toward the rescue, her in handcuffs, me walking next to her.

"Where are your parents?" I asked.

"They're dead!" she nearly screamed but was unable to get the necessary volume. It's tough to shout when your body just wants to cry. She was barely holding on to the tough facade.

I asked her if she would be okay during the ride to Hasbro Children's Hospital. She looked me in the eye, saw I could be trusted for now, and promised to be good. The police followed the rescue in their cruiser; the staff at the family counseling center went back to work.

She sat on the bench seat across from me while we rode. I started the state report while she stared at me.

"They didn't have to wreck my shoes," she said. Her flip-flops were thrown into the back of the truck after her, probably by one of the firefighters. I picked them up off the floor, put the good one on one foot, fixed the other one and put it on her other. Having something on my feet always makes me feel better, and it seemed to help Danielle. Maybe it took her mind off of being handcuffed.

"All better," I said.

"I wish," she responded and looked away. Tears started now. When all the rage is spent it's hard to keep them back, especially when you are fifteen years old.

"I want to go home with my mother," she sobbed. "I hate Woonsocket. I want to go home."

"Where is home?" I asked, not mentioning that she had said her parents were dead.

"Warwick. I just want to go home."

Our short-lived friendship ended when we arrived at Hasbro. The wall came up again, her game face back on. The tough girl returned, ready to battle anybody who got in her way.

I went back in service and got ready for the next call. I wish I could have done more.

Forgetting

Some looked happy, some sad, some looked at nothing at all. People are paid to watch them now, make sure they don't wander. After a lifetime watching their families grow, providing comfort, wisdom, direction, and roots, their role has diminished along with their vitality. Places like these have cropped up everywhere, an alternative to full-time nursing home care. It's not the best solution to a problem many families face, but it does provide safety and comfort for those whose lives have been shattered by Alzheimer's disease.

Our patient, a small, frail eighty-five-year-old lady, had been experiencing chest pain since the morning, I was told when I arrived on scene. She was in a private room away from the main activity room, a nurse, her daughter, and other staff members attending to her. They had given her a nitro tablet and told me all about the incident, how the pain began and radiated into her jaw and left arm. When I asked her she said her pain was seven out of ten on a one-to-ten scale.

Her vital signs were stable; we moved her onto our stretcher and wheeled her past her associates and into the bright sunshine. A minute later we were in the rescue, her on the stretcher, me on the bench. I asked her if the nitro pill had helped with her pain. She asked, "What pain?" I asked how she was feeling, she said, "A little tired, otherwise fine." She wanted to know what all the fuss was about.

I didn't know which story to believe.

Survivors
A couple in their early twenties went for a walk on Broad Street to get something to eat. Six guys mugged them, stole their McDonald's, roughed him up, then ran away. They were in the back of the rescue when the cops dragged one of the assailants over to be identified.

"That's him," they said, and the cops took the kid away. The guy's injuries weren't too bad—some bruises, a lump on the head; it could have been worse. Another young man was stabbed to death three blocks away a few nights ago while waiting to get into a popular nightspot. A girl was stabbed seven times last night and is still in critical condition. Try telling two kids whose dinner was just stolen by some punks that they are lucky, and they won't believe you. They were talking about getting a gun as we rode toward Rhode Island Hospital.

I Ain't Going!

"I ain't going to no hospital!"

"Yes you are."

"No, I ain't!"

"Yes you are."

"No I ain't!"

This was going well.

I was in the first-floor apartment of a diabetic seventy-year-old man. His skin was grey and diaphoretic, and blood oozed from untreated eczema in his crotch. He was conscious and alert but obviously in need of medical intervention. The guys from Engine 3 were in the tiny place with me and Vicro, the man's two daughters and a bunch of grandkids filled the kitchen and doorway.

One of his daughters called us because she was afraid for her father's well-being. He lived by himself, kept the place up fairly well, and was fiercely proud of his independence.

"I'm taking you to the hospital, even if I have to kidnap you."

"You and what army?"

I looked over to Rob Crellin, a firefighter from Engine 13 with a remarkable resemblance to Harry Potter.

"Me and Harry Potter."

Rob grabbed his right side, I took the left. We lifted him to his feet and started toward the stretcher. I couldn't believe the power that exuded from the tired old man's body. He stopped us in our tracks.

"I ain't going!" he shouted.

The man's family did their best to talk him in to going, but he adamantly refused. I refused to give up. This guy wouldn't make it through the night, I was sure of it.

"Let's go," I said to Rob. We picked him up and dropped him onto the stretcher, no nonsense this time. The strength he showed a few minutes ago was spent. He sat, rejected in the stretcher, as we strapped him in and wheeled him out of his home, maybe for the last time.

Once in the truck we took his vital signs. Blood pressure 64/40 with a pulse of 130. Possibly dehydrated, maybe internal bleeding. I felt his abdomen for point tenderness and masses, started a large-bore IV, and started fluids. The hospital was less than a mile away.

He ended up in a trauma room, more IVs, more fluids. Later that night I looked in on him. The doctor told me it was probably renal failure. Add that to his list of ailments. The man peeked at me through the labyrinth of wires and tubes and motioned for me to come closer. He offered his hand. I took it. In a low voice he said, "Thank you, boys. You knew what was best." He closed his eyes and went to sleep.

Kickball

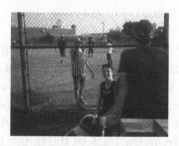

Just when I thought I had seen everything, the Providence Kickball League loses a player. She was running after a ball that had been kicked with abandon over her head when she fell forward, landing on her shoulder and possibly breaking her collarbone. Her teammates hovered over her while we immobilized her, first applying the cervical collar, then rolling her on her side and putting her onto the backboard. The opposing team, the Zombies, possibly extras from the *Night of the Living Dead* movie, stood to the side as the wounded player was removed from the field to the cheers of the large crowd that had gathered.

Fourteen teams belong to the league, mostly twenty-somethings having a ball. Or should I say, kick-ball. It seems like a great way to make friends, have some laughs, and stop taking ourselves so seriously. Play ball!

Fifty Days

The countdown has started. Fifty days until the 1207th finishes their time in Iraq.

"Hot, sand, and wind," is how Bob described his environment to me yesterday when he called. It still amazes me that he is in another world yet only a phone call away.

Keep your guard up, folks. You are in as much danger today as you were when you got there. Be safe and get home, all of you.

Ninety-Four

Amelia is ninety-four and has been taking her medication the same way for years and nobody, I mean NOBODY, is going to tell her different. We arrived at her home at 1034 hours. After knocking at the front door and not getting an answer, we went around the back. Meanwhile, Amelia was making her way from the back of the house to the front door. We knocked on the back door, no answer because Amelia had just struggled through her house to the front. I could hear cursing from inside. I had no idea what was going on at this point. I went back to the front door to see if I could pry it open, only now it was already open. I looked in and saw my patient walking back to the rear door. She moved pretty well for an older person.

I walked through the entryway past some stained-glass windows into a perfectly preserved fifties-style home. The workmanship was remarkable. Carved oak stairs, antique furniture that looked like it came off the showroom floor, a tile kitchen that would put today's workmen to shame. When I caught up with Amelia she was breathing fire.

"What's the matter?" I asked.

"These pills! I've been taking the same ones for forty years! I'm not taking these, they're not my pills!"

"Try to relax," I said, taking the prescription bottles from her hand. Our other five rescues were on other calls, surrounding cities and towns were responding into Providence on mutual aid, but I couldn't just leave her hanging. She was really upset.

After some consultation we found that her doctor couldn't be contacted, and the pharmacy had substituted her usual prescription with a generic type of the same medication. The dosage was different—she had to either cut the pills in half or take one every other day. She wasn't going for it, no way. The pharmacy went as far as sending a technician to her house to explain the situation. Nothing helped so she called 911, which is where we entered the picture.

I called the doctor's office and got stuck in the answering system, never connecting with a human. The message that stood out was, "If you are having an emergency, hang up and call 911," which is exactly what Amelia did. I called the pharmacy and talked to the pharmacist. This had been going on for two days, I was told. He promised to page the doctor and have him call Amelia. She refuses to take any medication until she hears from him.

She's ninety-four with a weak heart. The system is pushing her to her limit. I offered to take her to a hospital to get straightened out, but she refused. We did all we could do, which I'm afraid isn't enough.

Neighborhood Feud

"Rescue 1, respond to 25 Lennox Street for a pregnant female assaulted."

"Rescue 1, responding."

Vicro started the engine, hit the lights and siren, and sped out of the station toward our victim. It took four minutes.

"Rescue 1, on scene."

Engine 10 was parked in the middle of six of seven police cruisers. A crowd of fifty or so people wandered about, hurling threats at each other. The street was divided with us in the middle. Our patient sat on the cement steps in front of 25 Lennox looking totally out of place in all the madness. Lieutenant Dolan from Engine 10 gave me the story.

"She's twenty, was knocked to the ground, punched and kicked by two women."

I walked through the crowd of cops toward the victim. Things were under control, but barely.

"Can you check my baby?" the girl asked as I approached.

"We'll get you to the hospital so they can check you out," I replied, helping her to her feet. We walked back through the crowd toward the rescue. Once inside she told me what had happened.

"Four people with clubs and bats got out of that car," she said, pointing to a car through the rear windows of the rescue. "They knocked me over and kicked me in the stomach. One of them was on top of me, punching me." She didn't cry but was close. "Is my baby okay?"

Vicro had finished with the vitals, which were normal.

"I'm sure everything will be fine."

Some cops came in the side door and asked if she could identify the assailants. They indicated a woman standing next to the car behind the rescue with another police officer.

"That's the one who was sitting on me, punching me!" she said. She identified another; they were taken away in cuffs. We left the scene, which had become a circus. News people, onlookers, even the city councilman was there, giving an interview. The quicker we got away, the happier I was.

On the way to the hospital my patient talked. She is due on September 7 but hopes the baby waits until the tenth so she can finish her CNA class. She wants to be a pediatric nurse and is well on her way to reaching her dream. The people who attacked her were after her mother, she said, an old neighborhood feud. She just got in the way.

The people involved in the neighborhood feud just may get in the way of a girl from a rough neighborhood getting out.

No Escape

Monday night, all quiet. It had been a busy day, eleven or twelve runs since 0700, nothing serious, just enough to keep us rolling. At 2325 hours, Engine 6 got a call for a box alarm at one of the apartment buildings on Westminster Street. I couldn't believe my luck; I was certain I was going out when the tone went off and blow lights filled the station. I did the "ladder roll" when the lights went out and was instantly asleep. Seconds later, the phone rang. Once, twice, a half ring... Henry got it, lights out again. A minute later I was called to the apparatus floor. No rest for the wicked.

When Engine 6 left the barn, some asshat thought that the open door was his invitation to rummage around the station. Luckily, Chris Wright, who hours earlier had made perhaps the finest fajitas I have ever eaten, saw somebody enter the station before the door closed and called from the engine to warn us. When Henry got to the floor he saw a wiry Hispanic guy rummaging around the rescue. We shook him down—he didn't have time to steal anything—and tried to throw him out. The guy went into a crazy routine, acting like he was Jesus Christ and carrying on for a while before we grew tired of his act. Henry's prior employment at the Adult Correctional Institute (ACI) showed through as he handled the perpetrator perfectly. I radioed for the police when the guy started acting aggressive. A few minutes later a cruiser showed up and put the guy in the back of his car.

The guy was a street hood with a lengthy record who had just been released from prison in Ohio. His specialty was breaking and entering and robbery. In a strange twist of fate, his brother, also a cheap hoodlum, is recovering from stab wounds he got during a fight a few streets from the Hartford Avenue station. I think I had him in the rescue.

The cop took him away; we checked the locks and waited for the next call. I hate it when the sanctity of our station is invaded. This is our home when we're away from our families. It isn't perfect, but it's all we've got between us and them.

CHAPTER 12
AUGUST

Mercy

The fifteen floors of the Hartford Avenue housing projects loomed behind us as we walked through the oppressive late-night air toward our patient's apartment. She lived in a one-level unit, identical to others scattered about the area, some urban planners' good intentions gone bad. Broken glass and stale piss stuck to the bottoms of my shoes. I scraped them on the dew-covered crabgrass before walking through the doorway.

Screams came from somewhere inside, the words barely understandable but the anguish crystal clear. In the rear bedroom, lying on top of a filthy bare mattress in just her bra and panties, covered with sweat, we found the source of the screams.

"It hurts so bad!" she screamed over and over while clutching her belly. Fresh blood from under her panties joined whatever else lived on the mattress. "Get this baby out of me!" she cried.

We found out she was twenty-five weeks pregnant but hadn't felt the baby move in two days. Chris helped get her dressed, then moved her to the stair chair. We rolled her out of her place into the humid night air, screaming all the way. The ride to Women and Infants Hospital was no different; the only information I was able to get from her was that she had been shot in the back in 2004 and needed a colostomy bag. Her skin showed the scars of her ordeal between her tattoos.

At the hospital an ultrasound showed no movement. I left before finding out anything more, not proud of my thoughts at that moment. Henry and I didn't say much as we drove toward quarters. The night hadn't lifted the oppressive air from the city. Sunrise was upon us, things were already heating up.

Nobody Sleeps Tonight!

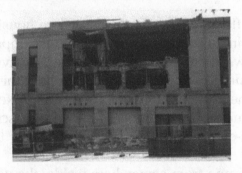

The hole in the middle of the LaSalle Square fire headquarters is where I spent my first night as a Providence firefighter. There, in the dorm, D-Boy told stories of fires and acts of heroism from his early years on the job, back in the sixties during the race riots when Providence burned. The reputation we now enjoy as one of the best departments in the country was forged during that era, back when three or four occupied house fires a night was common.

I lay in the bunk, ready wrapped, and listened as two guys from Special Hazards and Ladder 1, Jon Broom and Mike Keefe—who years later would fall some seventy feet from a broken tower ladder, ending the careers they loved—joined in the storytelling. Ranger Rick, Keith Edson, and Tony Toro from Engine 3 joined the banter, torturing each other, joking and filling the dorm with hysterical laughter. Keith (Gus) Grant and Sean Reddy, the other guys from Ladder 1, joined Bob Reilly from the Hazards, adding fuel to the fire until we made so much racket Captain Dillon stormed into the dorm, flipped on the lights, and announced, "NOBODY SLEEPS TONIGHT!"

Things were quiet for a while, then the bell tipped and I got my first taste of the red devil! While I dozed, Jon and Mike crumbled newspaper, put it on my bed, and set me on fire. Tony put me out with a bucket of water. The dorm went berserk again. Captain Dillon stayed away this time, probably afraid of what he would find. Lieutenant Cochrain from Engine 3 never left his room, but I can imagine him chuckling downstairs, knowing what the guys were putting me through.

Things quieted down again, but I stayed awake all night, soaked, smoky, and content. I've had a great career and expect more great years, but nothing will ever be as good as it was that night. I remember it like it was yesterday.

They can tear down the building, but the spirit of the firefighters who lived, who really lived, in that building will live forever.

The Wanderer
Things must have been dull at home so he went for a walk. Broad Street is a happening place. There's a bakery, a record store, people walking all over. Traffic moves fast but if you are quick you can get around without getting run over. Grandma took her pain pill and was asleep on the couch; TV was boring so off he went. Too bad the cops were on the ball; they ruined his stroll and took him home, six blocks away. What's a two-and-a-half-year-old supposed to do all day, watch his grandmother sleep?

Six Inches

Three years ago a young guy was killed while doing stunts with his motorcycle on Berkshire Street. He hit a fire hydrant while doing a wheelie. Every year his surviving friends and family gather around the hydrant to remember their loved one; a solemn, dignified moment in an inner city housing project.

Last night's memorial was interrupted when a van drove by the mourners, spraying them with gunfire, hitting two people and injuring more as they dove for cover. The brother of the motorcycle victim ended up in my rescue, his elbow shattered by a small-caliber bullet. Six inches to the left it would have been his heart. I took the kid's friend with us as we sped toward Rhode Island Hospital. They talked about how lucky they were to survive the ordeal, how chance plays such a huge role in determining who lives and who dies. A jump to the left instead of ducking when he saw the van approaching would have left him dead, his body full of holes instead of the building he stood in front of.

The emergency room was bustling with police activity when we arrived. There was a report of the shooters going to different hospitals to finish the job. Rhode Island Hospital was under intense police protection. Things seemed safe enough; I opened the rear doors of the rescue and brought my patients in.

Deported (departed)

"He's a diabetic," said one of the officers.

"I don't think that's the problem," I replied.

He was about to be deported. As soon as he arrived at the INS office his condition deteriorated, and within minutes he was seizing on the cement floor of the holding cell.

The guys from Engine 9 had an IV started and were working on vital signs.

"Let's get him in the truck."

As soon as I said it the guys lifted him from the floor and put him on the stretcher. We wheeled him out of the holding cell and past office staff and federal agents into the back of the reserve rescue we had for the day while Rescue 1 was out for repairs. Hot air blew from the air conditioning vents. I shut the AC off and we got to work in the hundred-degree heat.

"I need vitals and an EKG."

"I don't feel a pulse," said Mark

A flat line showed on the EKG screen. Shotzy checked the leads, Mark and Steve started CPR, Cappy got a vial of epinephrine ready. The patient remained pulseless, we pushed the epi, checked the screen, felt for a pulse; nothing.

We gave another round of epi, some atropine, continued CPR, tried and failed to intubate, and transported him to Rhode Island Hospital. I called the ER en route to give them time to get the trauma room ready. The team was assembled. The guys moved the patient from our stretcher to theirs, wires, tubes, IV bags, oxygen all sorted out in seconds. The room grew quiet, waiting to hear the story.

"Thirty-five-year-old in cardiac arrest, witnessed, diabetic history with a glucose of 134, seizure-like activity noted at 1605, asystolic upon EMS arrival at 1610, two rounds of epi, one atropine, two milligrams of Narcan, patient remains asystolic, CPR immediate upon arrest."

The trauma team got to work, started another IV, took over CPR, worked the code for fifteen minutes but never got a pulse.

Homecoming

Finally, Maria and Jeff brought John home. His crib at the ICU unit at Women and Infants Hospital was cozy enough. Pictures of the house, tractor, the dogs, and of course dad's fire truck made it bearable, but all the coming and going, wires, monitors, and racket made him eager to see home.

From all of us at Rescuing Providence (uh... me), welcome home!

Through the Haze

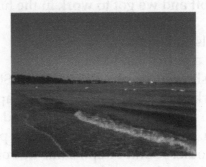

It never fails to amaze me when I travel this path how three miles separates the tranquil way of life I have grown accustomed to from the madness lurking on the horizon. The skyline of Providence can be seen in this picture, right in the middle, over the swans. My other life waits there, three days away. For now, I'll relax on the beach, watch the dogs bite the waves, and clear my head of last week's events.

News stories about one of my patients keep cropping up, his story and subsequent twisting of his sad demise a sorry indication of just how far off track our society has become. His body wasn't even cold before accusations of wrongdoing by the people sworn to uphold the laws of this great land were broadcast over the airwaves and in our newspapers. It's a wonder any of them bother to show up for work, knowing how eager the media is to hang them.

On another street, twenty hours later I tried and failed to revive a thirty-eight-year-old guy whose heart stopped after his pickup truck ran out of gas and he tried to push it up a hill. Nobody to blame for that one; no story to titillate the masses, no hot button issue to sell advertising, just another dead guy, younger than me, on the stretcher in back of my rescue.

A couple of kids got shot, a girl got beat up with a bat, another one hit by a car. Lonely old people needed someone to talk to, we were the only ones who listened. Drunks said they needed rehab, but only until their check came in and they could start all over.

I'll be starting over in a couple of days. From the beach I can see Providence through the haze, knowing that though I'm not there, it never really leaves me.

All for Nothing

The back of his head was smashed and there was a bump on his forehead. He had been drinking at the club, a place once full of wiseguys, now full of hot air. They showed him the door after getting him drunk, none too gently I'm sure.

"Why did they throw you out?" I asked.

"I'm not just an idiot . . . I work at it," he replied.

"What happened to your head?" I asked.

"Fell."

"Nobody hit you?"

"Fell."

He grew up on Federal Hill, in the heart of "Little Italy." In the sixties he would have been in his twenties, just the right age to be involved, or connected as we like to say around here. Raymond Patriarca was the man then, doing business from his office near where we found our patient. "Coin Vending" was all the sign outside said. I guess they couldn't fit extortion, prostitution, gambling, number running, drug dealing, and murder on it.

"I'm taking you to the hospital."

"I just want to go home."

"You're drunk and have a head injury. You're going to the hospital."

"Please, let me go home. I don't have insurance."

"They'll take care of you, don't worry."

He complained a little more but was in no position to argue. His blood pressure was 90/48, something seriously wrong besides the obvious. He talked a little about the old days, back when guys like him ran the city. Not having insurance would have been the least of his worries then. He wouldn't have been thrown out of the "club" either. They used to take care of their own. His arms showed prison tattoos, proof of time spent behind bars, probably for nothing more than keeping his mouth shut. Men didn't sing in those days. There was a twisted sense of honor among thieves.

As we approached the hospital he talked a little about the family. The fact that he was alone now, sick, old, and alone, didn't escape us. I asked if it was worth it.

"It was all for nothing," he said, dejected, and closed his eyes.

Rescue at Sea

The seven survivors were in the back of Rescue 1, shivering, laughing, and talking a mile a minute in Spanish. They had just survived a harrowing ordeal; their small boat had lost power in the Providence River and had run aground on the rocky, debris-filled shore of Fields Point. The guys from Engine 13 along with members of the Coast Guard secured a line to the boat and freed it from the abandoned pier where it was stuck. The guys looked like they had been fishing when trouble started.

We watched from the shore as their boat was towed toward safety with one of their party on board to man the wheel. Engine 13's taillights faded from view on land, the boat disappeared into the evening mist.

"What are we going to do with them?" one of the firefighters asked.

"Take them with me," I said.

"They won't fit."

"They fit in the boat."

One of them spoke English and told us where they parked their cars before launching. It was just across the river in East Providence.

"Pile in," I said while holding the rear doors of the rescue open. They fit.

When they tell their tale of misadventure to friends and family, I hope they mention the Providence Fire Department and US Coast Guard in a positive light. I know I enjoyed helping them.

Water Fire

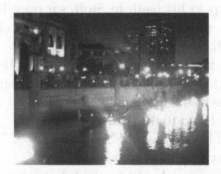

The light wind lifts the smoke from the river's surface and with it I feel my spirit rise. We leaned on the railing by the water's edge, my wife, Cheryl, by my side, soothing music hypnotizing the thousands in attendance as the gondolier rowed past. This is the heart of the city, not the streets where I spend most of my days. Here, a sense of peace and tranquility allows me to forget my troubles and focus on living. Not the living I have grown accustomed to, the lists, problems, and daily grind. This is the balance to that, when time stands still. I can focus on breathing, listening, and the sights around me.

Cold War

"What's your name?"

"Fuck you!"

"Is that your first or last name?"

"My name none of your business!"

"I thought it was fuck you."

"It's Mikhail Gorbachev!"

"Gorbachev is dead."

"So am I."

And so it went. We were called to one of the many high-rises in the city to take an intoxicated man to the hospital. Three police cruisers and one of our chief's cars were in front of the building when we arrived. An elderly Russian immigrant, up to his teeth in Stoli, sat on a bench outside cursing and pointing at the grim-faced officers. Chief Desmaris walked out of the lobby.

"This guy has been screwing with the elevators for an hour," he said. "He's got the place in an uproar."

It was three in the morning.

"Let's go," I said to the drunken man.

"Fuck you! I want lawyer!"

"I'm Johnny Cochran. Let's go."

"Johnny Cochran dead!" he said, but followed me to the truck anyway.

The ghosts of Gorbachev and Johnny Cochran rode to the hospital in the back of Rescue 1. It was a short ride. Gorbachev had settled down by the time we got there. We actually shared some laughs en route. I tried to tell him that the folks at the hospital won't tolerate any drunken behavior, but he didn't listen.

The party was over when I walked him into the ER and gave my report.

"Uncooperative, unknown male, intoxicated," I said to Marie and Alieda at triage. They had seen enough. As I walked back to the rescue, three security guards were descending on Gorbachev, restraints ready.

Take Your Runs!
We try, we really do, to keep up with the calls that keep coming. One after the other people call, sometimes all at once. Six rescues for a city the size of Providence is simply not enough.

There are times when you just can't take another one. Fatigue, frustration, and hunger all contribute to turning a deaf ear to the radio. Somehow, the obvious "true" emergencies get through, the stubbed toes, toothaches, etc., all turn into static when you have had enough.

Wednesday night, midnight. Rescue 1 was called to Charles Street for a man who "couldn't sleep." Charles Street is in the heart of Rescue 3's area. I listened to the radio for a minute, silently praying I would hear the lieutenant from Rescue 3 come in service and take his run. No such luck. Most of the shift was working overtime, everybody was shot. One more, I thought, and out the door we went.

Interstate 95 was closed due to the construction project, so we had to go through the city. There wasn't much traffic at this hour, only one vehicle ahead of us. Could it be? You bet. Rescue 3. We passed them, lights and sirens blaring, except for when we turned off the siren to say "Take your runs!" over the PA system. Had I not been guilty of similar infractions in the past I might have been mad; instead, I found the whole situation hilarious. They would have pulled it off had the on ramp been open. There is an art to deception, but it takes years of practice.

Rescue 3's officer, name deleted at the officer's request, got on the radio a minute later and offered to take the call.

"Negative, fire alarm, we're a few feet ahead of him, we'll continue," I said over the air. I could hear the dispatcher's chuckle in the background. They all know the intricate chess game we play on the streets while trying to maintain our sanity.

A few minutes after we arrived at Charles Street, Rescue 3 got a call for an intoxicated man in Olneyville. Rescue 6 didn't surface; the 3s took the call.

Another night in Providence.

Used to Be My Chair

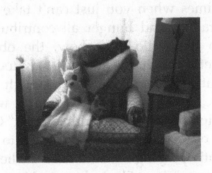

Friends

Rescue 1 rolled into the rescue bay at Rhode Island Hospital at around ten o'clock. Zack and Teresa opened the side and rear doors simultaneously as we sometimes do to say hello and see if we can help. My patient was an eighteen-year-old kid who looked healthy enough, unless you had just heard her story. I said hello to Zack and Teresa and walked through the doors with Monica.

"What's wrong?" Teresa asked.

"Nothing, just tired."

I wasn't tired and Teresa knew it. She stayed outside with Zack and the other guys, catching up on the latest gossip and getting ready for more runs. It's a ritual we all look forward to. One by one the rescues leave, either going on calls or just heading back to the station.

I gave my report to the triage nurses, glad that it was Katy working, somebody I knew would take good care of the patient.

"She's eighteen, complaining of pain to her lower abdomen, bruises to the right side of her face, lumps on the back of her head and neck. She was forcibly raped in Boston, didn't know what to do, got on a bus and came here. We're the first people she's talked to, the police are on their way."

Katy walked over to Monica, crouched down so she was at eye level, and started to talk to her. My job was done, so I went back outside. Zack and Teresa were still there.

I told them about the girl. They understood my somber mood and didn't push for any more. I got back in the truck and headed back to the station.

I saw them a few hours later, same place, only I was back to normal.

Twenty-One Days and a Wake-Up

Their replacements are straggling in, twenty today, some more tomorrow. Soon the entire 1207th will be replaced by the "new guys." Twenty-one days left. Stay safe, folks!

It's been well over a year since they reported for training last July. A lot has happened during that time. Here, at home we continued to build our careers, watched our children grow, planted gardens and enjoyed the fruits of our labor, enjoyed the pleasure of our spouse's company, and gotten on with our lives.

There, they have eaten sand and sweat, followed orders, gave orders, seen friends get hurt and die, and watched as the world moved on without them. There are no tomato gardens in the desert. There are bullets and bombs and people who want to kill us. Thank you, Bob, and everybody from the 1207th and everybody else over there for standing in their way. Your sacrifices are almost done, but what you have accomplished will never be forgotten, not by me or anybody else who calls themselves an American.

Ultimate Sacrifices
Two Boston firefighters paid the ultimate sacrifice last night. Two New York firefighters last week. Rest in peace, brothers, we'll see you in Heaven. Condolences to their families.

Life Moves Fast
Stubborn old coot got his leg stuck under the front seat of the van he was trying to get into. Instead of sending a sedan like they usually do, the cab company sent the minivan. Dan should have waited, at least that's what his wife of fifty-eight years said as she stood under a shade tree a few feet away and watched us work. They had moved into the place only a week and a half ago, she said. They had to give up their home in Cranston, just couldn't keep it up. They were worried about their failing health as well. It looked as though they found a nice place to enjoy some quiet years.

Dan had maneuvered himself so he was kneeling on one knee but the other leg just got "more stuck." The more he moved, the "more stuck" it got. He was howling in pain when we arrived. The assisted living staff, the cabbie, Dan's wife, some neighborhood kids—all were helpless, waiting for somebody who knew what to do.

Call 911! I thought as I looked at the hopelessly stuck leg. *You ARE 911!*

Better think of something. I tried to move the seat forward, Dan's howling intensified. Plan B. I had Veakro lift from one side while I lifted him from the other, trying to get him back to a forward position. No go. I thought I had ripped his leg off from the noise he made. From my vantage point there was no bleeding, no deformity, and no way we were going to get him out of there without making a huge production out of this, hydraulic equipment, Special Hazards, the whole nine yards.

"Veakro, on three," I said. Veakro understood. He grabbed one arm and leg, I grabbed the other.

"One, two, THREE!"

We lifted, turned, and weaseled him out from under the seat in about three seconds. He stopped shouting once his leg was free. We helped him stand up, put pressure on the leg, and take a few steps. I wanted to take him to the ER for an evaluation; he said he had called for a cab to get to his doctor's appointment. He was proud of his independence. He signed a refusal form and we said good-bye . . .

Midnight. A call came in to the same address for a man bleeding from the head in an assisted living facility, the same one where we helped Dan earlier in the day. Sure enough, we opened one of the apartment doors and there was Dan, a six-inch laceration to the top of his head, lying in a pool of blood on the bathroom floor, his wife standing next to him. He was nearly unconscious but looked at me all the way to the hospital. He suffered a stroke, then fell to the floor, smashing his head.

A week and a half. From homeowners, to assisted living, and now, in all likelihood, a nursing home.

Life moves fast as you get older.

CHAPTER 13
SEPTEMBER

Helmets

He could have been my brother or friend or a guy I work with. If not for the drool dripping from the corner of his mouth and helmet he wore on his head, he looked like your typical thirty-eight-year-old guy. He lived with people three times his age, sick, dying people in need of constant medical supervision. I wondered how he ended up in a nursing home. The interagency report I read as we rode toward Rhode Island Hospital didn't tell me much, only that he refused to take his medication because it was crushed in applesauce and was threatening the other patients and staff. He didn't look very menacing to me, but then I'm not ninety years old and confined to a wheelchair or bed.

"What are you doing living in a nursing home?" I asked, not knowing if he was capable of answering. He pointed to his head.

"What's wrong with your head?"

"Motorcycle." He slurred the word the best he could.

"Accident?" I asked. He shook his head yes.

"Were you wearing a helmet?"

He pointed to the helmet on his head.

"Am now."

I found out later he had suffered massive head injuries as

a result of a motorcycle accident four years ago. His Harley was ruined when somebody pulled out of a side street in front of him. He wasn't going that fast, maybe forty, but fast enough to land him in a nursing home being spoon-fed medication for the rest of his life, his only excitement acting up and scaring the old folks.

Some days I think I have things pretty much figured out. Days like this I just look at my patient, shake my head, and wonder.

Valium, Vicodin, and Nachos
Eventually, carrying people up and down stairs and into and out of the rescue takes its toll. Last week I felt something give. I've been hobbling around for about ten days now; back injury. It happened while transporting a twenty-five-year-old patient from her OBGYN's office to the emergency room at Women and Infants Hospital. The buildings are connected; the patient could have been transported to the ER by hospital staff in less than five minutes without ever leaving the building. Instead, the person in charge of the patient at the doctor's office decided that 911 was the best way to transport the patient, noncritical, contractions about eight minutes apart, no complications.

I digress. Pent-up frustration at the abuse of the 911 system, I guess.

"Fat, drunk, and stupid is no way to go through life, son," the dean told Kent "Flounder" Dorfman in *Animal House*.

Valium, Vicodin, and nachos aren't much better. I'll be off the couch in a few days. I'm looking forward to getting back to work.

Never Forget
The president of Local 799, Paul Doughty, asked me to be the keynote speaker at this year's 9-11 memorial service at

police and fire headquarters. It was short notice, but I put the following words together just in time. I thought I would share them with you.

It is vitally important that we come together on this date to honor those who lost their lives on September 11, 2001. It's hard to believe, but six years have passed. The memorials have grown smaller, the painful memories easier to bear. Some people prefer to block it from their minds, act as if it never happened. That's their choice, not ours. Time marches on; new experiences take place of memories we once thought would be with us forever. From the depths of sorrow, we find hope. It's a good and necessary thing. Without it we would be crushed by the weight of sorrow that builds as the years go by.

We've learned to live with the painful memories from that day, but we will "never forget!" It's up to us to keep the memory of the fallen alive. This isn't just another day. It's a day when every American, especially firefighters, needs to stop and think of what we have, those who fight for it, those who died protecting it, and vow to keep their memory alive.

Never forget that every time we put our gear in the truck, we honor the memory of the 343 firefighters who died while doing their job six years ago. Every one of us knows we may be asked to risk everything while doing our job. It's not heroic or glamorous or anything else we may have thought it was before we took the oath. It's simply what we do. We are born with it; it's in our blood. Some see it as a curse; most consider it a blessing.

The firefighters that died that day were people like us, proud of their profession, their families, and their ability to save lives and protect property. I'm sure there was a little swagger in their walk that morning when they started their shift, confident they could handle anything thrown at them and somehow walk away. We think the same way; if we didn't, we wouldn't be wearing these uniforms. But with that swagger comes a price. People expect us to save them, and we usually do. Sometimes we don't, and sometimes we die with them.

Thousands of regular citizens showed up for work that day, entered the elevators, sat at their desks, talked at the water cooler, and got prepared to start their day. Nothing could have prepared them for what happened next. Most of those that weren't killed instantly waited. For us. We responded. As the world watched the drama unfold on their televisions, helplessly, we responded.

If they thought the job hopeless, they never would have tried it. They thought there was a chance, and they marched to their deaths. They didn't go to work that day expecting to die. None of us go to work expecting to die. Ours is a different profession. We take risks. We work hard and punish our bodies, not because we have a death wish; rather, we have a wish that we can make things right when they go horribly wrong, as they did on September 11, 2001. Those who entered the towers thought the poor souls on the upper floors had a chance and they went to go get them.

When the first tower fell, I knew. Before the top floor hit the ground, I said to my wife, "We just lost a lot of firefighters."

"Why were they still in there?" she asked."

"They were doing their job."

She looked at me, shook her head, and looked back at the TV, knowing if I were there, I would have been in the tower. It's harder on our families than it is on us.

We owe it to the firefighters who died that day to keep getting on that truck and doing our best, whether it's in New York City, Providence, Warwick, or Cumberland, and to keep doing what they did six years ago for them the final time: our duty.

I learned an important lesson that day and the weeks and months to follow. The people we are sworn to protect are worth protecting. We stood together as a nation like nobody could have dreamed possible. We remembered what it meant to be Americans; we stood together, cried together, and together have moved forward. Racial and economic divisions didn't matter, differing political philosophies were irrelevant.

In many ways we've returned to our pre-911 mindset, and that is unfortunate, but the togetherness and resolve that existed then still resides in all of us, and comes to the surface when necessary. I know it's there. I remember, and that is what keeps me going.

It's good to be alive, and an honor to be part of the Providence Fire Department and member of Local 799, but most of all, it's good to be a firefighter.

Fifteen

Body language, facial expressions, a few common words spoken are usually enough. So young, I thought, holding my index finger and thumb as if holding a card. She reached into her purse and produced an ID. It was a Guatemalan embassy card. The language barrier was easily overcome, the worlds that separated us impossible to breach.

Even if I knew how to say it, I wouldn't give her the same speech saved for my own child. She smiled radiantly and looked at me as I filled out the report. Any wisdom I had to share with her I kept to myself. What to one child is a bad decision is a lifesaver to another. If this were my daughter, I would tell her she had the rest of her life ahead of her, friends, dates, proms, graduation, college, career, and a world to conquer.

I smiled back at the fifteen-year-old girl sitting across from me. Her future grew inside of her, thirty-seven weeks along. Anchor babies, some people call them.

Snoring

He lay crumbled at the bottom of a cement stairway, his head at an odd angle, snoring. There are drunk snores, fake snores, sound asleep snores, and snores like this one; a get him on oxygen, immobilized, extricated, IV'd, monitored, medicated, and to the trauma room snores.

We've done this thousands of times. The patient was in the trauma room ten minutes later, the operating room half an hour after that. The people I work with are truly the best around. Engine 3 assisted on scene, the Rhode Island Hospital trauma team took over, then the operating room crew from there. He'll probably end up in the intensive care unit, then a "regular room" and hopefully some therapy, home care, and with a little luck full recovery.

Or, he could never regain consciousness and all of our work will be for nothing.

Unexpected Jolt

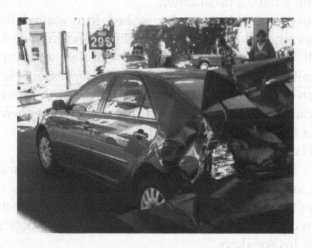

This guy's coffee had a little extra "kick" this morning. He had stopped to get a cup of joe and say hello to some friends; when he got back into his car with his coffee another car clobbered him. A few months ago a nineteen-year-old kid was hit in this exact spot so hard he was thrown from the rear window and killed. My patient was lucky, minor injuries. We secured him on a spine board, applied a cervical collar, and transported him to the Rhode Island Hospital emergency room.

The neighbors formed a posse and found the alleged driver about a mile away, inside a coffee shop, having a coffee. The cops told me later the man was heavily intoxicated.

Don't people go to church on Sundays anymore?

No Help Here

We've got a problem. Mentally ill patients have nowhere to go. It's a catch-22 situation; those with the most severe problems cannot keep jobs and have no insurance. Cuts in state spending have reduced the number of "uninsured" beds in the area hospitals. These folks have nowhere to go when they have a breakdown.

A fifty-year-old guy who looked forty called for help this morning. They said he had a knife and intended to kill himself. The police arrived first and found no weapon, so we were called in. The man was obviously depressed. He sat on the curb in front of a dilapidated house in South Providence. The house needed to be razed and rebuilt but there were signs of life there. I asked him if he lived there.

"I wish."

He's been staying in homeless shelters for years, can't keep a job, can't afford the psych meds that could help him, and can't find a reason to go on living. He's been incontinent for two days now, the evidence clinging to the bottom and sides of his sneakers.

"Get in the truck," I said. Al put some extra sheets on the stretcher and we got moving.

"I just can't hold it anymore," he told me when I asked about the mess.

He stared blankly at the ceiling as we rode toward Rhode Island Hospital. There he will be given a psych evaluation. If he is lucky he will be given a bed and proper treatment in a psych ward somewhere—Kent Hospital, Butler, or the Jane Brown Building at Rhode Island Hospital. More likely he will be put into the clinical decision unit at the emergency room until he is cleared. That could take days. The lights never go out; the space is shared with the dozens of intoxicated persons we take in from the streets. He'll be forced to lie in bed and listen to the madness that surrounds him. If he breaks and gets overactive or vocal he will be restrained.

I wanted to help this man get back on his feet. Instead, I delivered him to the door of more madness.

Al knew what I was feeling after we brought him in.

"What are you going to do?" he asked, shaking his head, knowing there was no answer.

"Rescue 1 in service," I said into the mic, and we rolled back into the city.

Taint

I was a little disappointed to find my patient alert, conscious, and ambulatory. There was some blood spattered on a kitchen chair. A lady with a bucket and mop smiled at me and finished washing the floor. Not quite the scene I had envisioned during the five-minute response time. We were dispatched for a severe upper leg laceration from a power saw. Don't get me wrong, I don't want to see anybody lose a limb or bleed to death, but it is a letdown once you have yourself prepared for the worst.

My patient was an affable nineteen-year-old who was helping his uncle renovate their hundred-year-old home. Places like this are sprouting up everywhere I look, little gems in the desert. A freshly painted fence adorned with colorful mums led us into the place. Emelio, the wounded worker, was putting on a robe in another room while we waited. The uncle took off his tool belt and waited with us.

"Did you do these floors?" I asked.

"Southern yellow fir," he said, proudly. "You can't buy this now, all gone."

I had the same flooring in my last house, beautiful stuff, once refinished.

"Your place is looking good," I complimented him. They had done a lot of work. When they finished it would add value to the entire street. Soon, I hope, the rundown places will be out of place here. Pride of ownership does a lot for a neighborhood.

Emelio limped out of a bedroom and walked to the truck, his uncle coming along.

"What happened?" I asked.

"I sat on a nail. It bled for a while but it's stopped."

"Where is the puncture?"

He looked miserable, trying to explain. It must have been embarrassing to a nineteen-year-old kid.

"It's kind of at the top of my leg, uh . . . kind of near my . . . umm, testicles, but a little behind . . . umm . . ."

"Did you puncture your anus?"

"No, a little behind." The poor kid was squirming, didn't know what to say.

"Oh, your taint," I said and started the report. He looked confused, but relieved.

His uncle asked, "What's a taint?"

"It ain't your balls and it ain't your ass. Taint." I shrugged my shoulders like this happened every day and kept on writing.

They almost fell out of the truck laughing. Nothing like a little male bonding to set things straight.

Nice Day

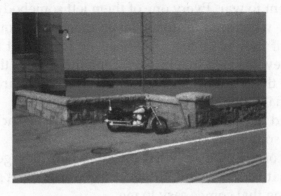

I rode past my brother's house today, forgot the kids are all in school. Beautiful day for a ride anyway. A couple of waterfalls, windy country roads, little or no traffic, and the smell of late summer woods to keep me company. I had to stop and take a picture here; a quick shot from my phone isn't as good as a panoramic view of the Scituate Reservoir from the middle of the bridge, but it's better than nothing. Bob will be home in a week and a couple of days. Can't wait.

Sorry, Bro, but you can't have your bike back. You survived Iraq, I'd hate to see you get hurt on your motorcycle, so for your own good, I'm keeping it!

Piling On

The next time I complain about my back I'll remember Serena. Fifty-seven years old, pretty face, nice family, room full of good books and movies and a few other things. Congestive heart failure, COPD, renal failure, diabetes, left leg amputated, cancer, gangrene, chronic nausea and vomiting, to name a few. She smiled between gasps for air on the way to the hospital. The strength of the human spirit endures, and makes my minor pains just an annoyance.

Soldiers

They went to war. Every one of them left somebody behind, someone who cared for them, loved them, and would never recover if they were lost. They had no idea what to expect when they boarded that bus last September, only that some, or all of them might not come back. Well, they are coming back. Finally, they're on their way home.

Behind the hugs and handshakes, pats on the back, and all that lies something deeper.

"Welcome home" is what I'll say when they get off the bus. What I feel I know I'll never say out loud. It's just not something that comes easy to me.

You stood tall, conquered your fears, did your job and did it well. You endured months of loneliness in a hostile desert, saw things that will haunt your dreams forever. You did what was right, not because somebody told you to, but because you said you would do what it takes when you joined the Guard. You were good to your word.

Nobody can take that away from you. For the rest of your lives you will carry with you the memories. Some people may forget what you did, but those are the ones who never cared to begin with. They wouldn't stand up for themselves in times of trouble. You stood up for them and the rest of us, and for that, those of us who do care are forever grateful.

Things haven't changed much since you were gone. We've aged a year, and so have you. Something grew during that time. Something that can't be seen unless you look closely. People will never look at you the same way again. You may not feel differently, but we will see you in a different light. We'll see what you are — valiant soldiers who have earned our respect.

Enjoy it. Few deserve it, most will never experience it, but you will wear it for as long as you live.

Thank you, Brother, and all the members of the 1207th Transportation Company of the Rhode Island National Guard. Welcome home.

Men of Providence

We had a rash of wife beaters last night, three in a row between ten and midnight. An eighteen-year-old girl was hit in the head with a baseball bat; she was dazed but conscious. When we arrived on scene she was holding a ten-month-old infant, swaying from side to side, barely able to stay seated. She handed the baby off to her brother and came with us to the hospital. Twenty minutes later, a few blocks away another girl ran from her home, broken cell phone in her hand, new wounds included pain in her chest from being kicked, a lacerated nostril from where her nose ring used to be before her "boyfriend" ripped it out, and abdominal pain from more kicks. Bruises covered her arms legs, and torso, evidence of months of abuse. Another girl was found standing on Broad Street with no shoes bleeding from her mouth. Her boyfriend punched her in the face and threw her out.

Together Again

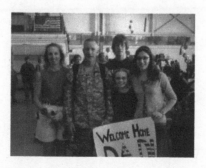

As soon as the two C-130 transport planes appeared on the horizon, the crowd erupted. Families, friends, politicians, the

Patriot Guard; everybody cheered. Flags waved as the planes roared overhead. They banked sharply left and rolled out of sight. A minute later one, then the other taxied past us on the runway. In perfect precision they turned, faced us, and stopped. It was truly beautiful. The soldiers disembarked, stood in formation for a minute, then joined their families. It was a perfect moment. I took this picture and left. I'll catch up tomorrow.

The people fighting this war are an incredible group of people. I'm proud to know them.

CHAPTER 14
OCTOBER

Pedestrian Struck

The guys from Ladder 8 were cleaning her head wound and getting ready to apply a cervical collar when we arrived on scene. A good amount of blood spattered the ground and the victim's clothing. She was awake but stunned, sitting in the road in front of an older Toyota.

You never know what to expect when dispatched for a pedestrian struck. The injuries could be life threatening, disfiguring, or extremely painful. Broken bones, lacerations, and concussions are common. This patient didn't look to be hurt too badly. She didn't lose consciousness and there were no gross deformities. The only problem I could see was the head injury. There was no damage to the Toyota.

We put her on the spine board and loaded her onto the stretcher, then into the rescue. She had just stepped out of her car when she was hit. As Veakro checked her vitals I gathered the necessary information.

"I don't have insurance," she said, worried.

"Don't worry, the person who hit you will have insurance, they'll pay the bill."

"Bicycle riders need insurance?"

I looked out the side window of the rescue. Next to her Toyota a bicyclist talked to the police, his front tire bent.

You never know what to expect.

Flashback

Desperate people sometimes do desperate things. A thirty-year-old guy with a drug problem found a new way to feed his habit. The high-voltage power lines that bring electricity from the power plants up north are secured in place by guy wires. The material is expensive, even as scrap metal.

Somehow, one of the guy wires let loose and contacted the live wires, electrocuting the man trying to steal them. Neighbors heard the "pop" and saw the flash from a half mile away. He tried to crawl up the embankment to get help after trying his cell phone, only to find it had melted. Somebody called 911.

I was at Rhode Island Hospital talking to Jeff Davenport, who was detailed in charge of Rescue 2 for the day. My truck wasn't ready; Rescue 2 took the call as I listened on the radio. Lieutenant Mike Clark and Engine 12 were first on scene.

"Engine 12 to fire alarm, we have a young adult with third-degree burns over 90 percent of his body, possible live wires in the area, have companies use extreme caution."

Special Hazards arrived on scene and secured the area, the electric company was called in, Battalion 2 took over as the incident commander. I'm not sure how, but they got the patient away from the immediate danger and into Rescue 2. His skin had melted. Matt, Rescue 2's chauffeur, told me later his uniform was covered with the patient's skin.

If the patient has any chance of survival he owes it to the firefighters who responded. Woody from Ladder 1 spent eight or nine of his seventeen years on the job in the rescue division. Dave from Engine 12 is a skilled EMT C with extensive rescue experience. Lieutenant Clarke is an RN, Matt is a paramedic. Somehow they started an IV, kept the patients skin intact, provided oxygen, and got him to the trauma room at Rhode Island Hospital in about fifteen minutes.

This incident could have happened anywhere in the city, on any group at any time, and people with similar training and expertise would have responded. Everybody plays a part, everybody performs above and beyond what is considered by anybody's standards exceptional. The people of Providence are well served by their firefighters.

I worked overtime at Rescue 2 that night. As I sat at the desk waiting for Jeff to return from another call I started to do some reports for him. The third one down had a familiar scent. I read the report; it was the burn victim's, the smell of his flesh embedded into the paper. It was a haunting experience. Memories of incidents I thought long forgotten flashed through my mind as I got up and walked out of the room, looking for some fresh air.

Communication Breakdown

Just when I think I speak enough Spanish to get by, somebody throws me a curve.

0200 hours; an intoxicated man on Westminster Street. He's a Guatemalan immigrant, pleasant enough, obviously inebriated and unable to find his way home. I thought he was too drunk to speak, turns out he is mute. He was a whiz at sign language; all the way to the hospital he signed messages to me.

I didn't understand a word he signed.

Knuckleball

Just when I've got the curve figured out, somebody brings in the knuckleballer! 1130 hours, called for an unresponsive thirty-eight-year-old male. Arrived on scene and found a guy lying in bed, unconscious, unresponsive, respirations 6/minute, strong pulse, 110/72 with pinpoint pupils. Everything pointed toward heroin overdose.

I administered 2 mg Narcan IM immediately, had Jay assist ventilations as the guys from Engine 13 got ready to move him. We got him onto the stair chair and into the rescue in about four minutes. During that time he began to respond to the Narcan. His breathing improved but was nowhere near normal. He did open his eyes when I gave him a sternal rub. Jay continued to bag him, Steve and Veakro started an IV, and we gave him two more milligrams of Narcan. A minute later he was conscious but still not alert and unable to communicate with us. He still had trouble breathing and started to panic.

As we got ready to transport to Rhode Island Hospital, another man showed up. He couldn't communicate either; he and the man on the stretcher were brothers, both born deaf and living together. Through rudimentary sign language and gestures we were able to put together some pieces of the puzzle as we rode toward the hospital.

A few hours later I looked in on them. The brother who had overdosed was intubated and in the intensive care unit, probably suffering with pneumonia as well as the aftereffects of the OD. His brother stood vigil outside the door, waiting for something good to happen.

Book Release
My friend Ann Martini from Wright Martini Media thought it would be a good idea to have a book release party when *Rescuing Providence* was published. Never one to pass on an opportunity for a party, I agreed. Not knowing what to expect, we planned for a few weeks. Ann's husband, Michael, prepared the food, Brittany was the bartender, Danielle passed out hors d'oeuvres, Ann handled the million little details, and my wife, Cheryl, added her personal touch with a few dishes of her own as well as organizing the book signing part of things.

My thanks to them all for making it possible.

I am still overwhelmed with the outpouring of support from my family, friends, coworkers, and some new acquaintances.

Well over a hundred people showed up. It was a gratifying, memorable, and ultimately humbling moment for me. Gaining and keeping the respect of those closest to me is not something I take lightly. It has given me a fresh perspective, no small amount of pride and accomplishment, and a great amount of satisfaction. For that I am truly thankful.

If everybody enjoys the book one tenth as much as I enjoy knowing them, I will consider it a success.

Greatest Generation

He's eighty-two, a WWII veteran, lying on the floor of his dirty one room apartment in Olneyville, his piss bag nearly full, his left arm broken. At some time during the night he fell out of his wheelchair and couldn't get up. By the time we got there he was nearly delirious. Pain, dehydration and fear mixed together with loneliness and despair must have made for an awful night. We wrapped his arm the best we could, lifted him onto our stretcher, locked his door and took him away.

Code Red!

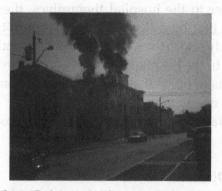

Fire on Blain Street. Took our guys about twenty minutes to bring it under control. Great job!

Breeders

Yesterday a twenty-four-year-old, eighteen weeks pregnant person called 911 from just outside the parking lot of Women and Infants Hospital because she was nauseous. We were at Miriam Hospital, the other end of Providence. No other rescues were available, so we took the run. Traffic, road construction, and drivers who didn't give a hoot that there was an emergency vehicle trying to get through contributed to a ten minute response time. We arrived on scene, helped the "patient" into the truck. She sat on the bench seat and projectile vomited all over the stretcher, floor, and my shoes. No warning or apology, or even the slightest remorse. Thirty seconds later we walked her into Woman and Infants Hospital, where she informed the triage nurse she "felt much better" now that she had vomited and didn't need to be seen.

A few hours ago, another pregnant female felt pain in her side while at work. She called her family to come get her, the pain too much to bear. They drove to her place of employment, put her into their car, drove back to their home, past Women and Infants Hospital, and into their driveway. After helping her into their home, they called 911. When I asked why they didn't take her to the hospital themselves, they indignantly informed me that by calling 911 they wouldn't have to wait with everybody else in the waiting room. Her vitals were stable; we drove her to the hospital, where she joined everybody else. I asked the triage nurse if she could put her name behind the people who came in after her.

Another day breeding responsible citizens here in the capital city.

Lunchtime Disaster

He left his daughter's home in Warwick at 11:30. They were going to have lunch together; Chinese takeout. At 12:30 his daughter called the Warwick Police, concerned that her diabetic father hadn't returned. At 12:45 we received a call for a pedestrian struck by an auto. Approaching the scene I saw not one, but two separate incidents:

A young man sitting next to his banged-up bicycle, holding his knees to his chest, and

A mid-sized car that had driven through a chain-link fence and into the side of a brick building.

As we approached, Lieutenant Mahoney told me that the person in the car was more critical than the man next to the bike. He had already called for an additional rescue; I went to the car and took a look inside.

The driver was about seventy years old, sitting in the driver's seat, no seat belt, and unconscious. A metal fence pole pierced the windshield, barely missing the driver's head as it swept through the passenger compartment. The car tipped dangerously on its side. The guys from Engine 13 declared the scene safe, so me and Mark, my driver for the day, opened the driver's side door and extricated the victim. He was unresponsive at first, and then started to struggle. There was no evidence of alcohol; I assumed it was a diabetic emergency. We got him into the rescue; vital signs, IV, oxygen, and a blood glucose test in about a minute. His glucose level was 40. An amp of D-50 later our patient had regained consciousness.

He told me he left his daughter's house in Warwick to get some lunch at the Chinese takeout and couldn't remember anything after leaving her driveway. He didn't remember getting onto the highway, driving nearly ten miles, taking an exit into Providence, running down a guy on a bicycle, tearing through a fence, and smashing into a brick building. I found his cell phone in his pocket, saw seven missed calls from Monica. I hit the send button, Monica answered on the first ring. She was relieved that her dad was okay but concerned for the well-being of the man on the bicycle. Luckily, that guy was only shaken up.

We transported him to Rhode Island Hospital, one very lucky guy.

That Hurt!
Well, I'm feeling pretty darn good about myself. My party was a smashing success, the job is going well, my friends and family think I'm some big shot author, and my book is being displayed at Borders bookstore on the register table right next to one of my favorites, Bruce Springsteen's newest CD.

I figured I would share my success with Megan, a very pretty twenty-four-year-old nursing student and Rhode Island Hospital employee.

"Me and Springsteen have something in common," I told her after telling her about my book and its prominent spot at Borders.

"I know," she said, dead serious. "You're both old."

It's good to be back on earth. Thanks, Megan!

No Help
I learned what little Spanish I know because there was a need to communicate with my patients. It's easy to say, "Speak English!" It's not as easy when the person speaking Spanish is dying in front of you while their family looks on helplessly, unable to communicate. Simple phrases such as "what is your name, when were you born, where is your pain, how bad is it, when did it start, do you take medications, do you have allergies to medications" are easy to learn and help ease tension during an emergency.

If I can learn a little Spanish, there is absolutely no excuse for people living in this country not to make an attempt to learn some English.

Friday night, 0300. We got a call for a woman with chest pain. We arrived at her home, a well-kept one-story in a terrible neighborhood surrounded by an ornate fence, three $30,000 and up cars in front and in the driveway, marble tile floors, beautiful furniture and paintings, and a fifty-eight-year-old lady sitting on the couch clutching her chest, Five family members surrounded her. I tried to communicate with my limited Spanish; they made no effort to help. Four firefighters looked on as we tried everything to communicate with these people, but they couldn't convey their message.

"What is your name?" I asked in Spanish. She did answer that.

"Are you in pain?" Yes.

"When did it start?" No answer there, just a lot of chatter from the family that I didn't understand.

"Where are your medications?" You would think I asked them to recite the Constitution. Nobody moved.

After more noncommunication, I assumed she was having chest pain with a history of heart problems. She couldn't stand up. We carried the woman to the truck, 350 pounds, five feet four inches. She carried on the entire time. The family followed us in one of their expensive cars.

We did an IV, gave her a nitro, aspirin, and oxygen, ran an EKG, and transported her to Rhode Island Hospital. There, a Spanish interpreter told us that the woman witnessed her daughter and her daughter's boyfriend have an argument and she was upset. No chest pain, no history, just "upset."

I was pretty upset myself. I think I'll learn how to say that in Spanish.

Ortega Like the Sauce

"What happened?"

"Yo, like this bitch stone cold upped me."

"She what?"

"My bike, bro, I'm chillin sho holed me up, bro."

"What are you talking about?"

"I need medication, give me some Vicodin."

"Are you nuts?"

"Take me home, bro, just give me some Vicodin."

"I'm taking you to the hospital."

"Yo, don't go without my halfbelt, it's flyin' on the ground."

Sure enough, there on the ground was half a belt. I always wondered how they kept their pants halfway on their body.

"What's you name?"

"Emelio Ortega, like the sauce."

"Have you been drinking, Emelio Ortega Like the Sauce?"

"Two beers, bro, I'm twenty-one. Just take me home, bro, I need some Vicodins and my crib, I'll be chillin'."

We took him to Rhode Island Hospital, where he tortured Kris and Ron for a while. I have no idea what his problem was other than he was riding his bike and "some bitch stone cold upped" him.

Stop Crying!

Ten months old, permanent brain damage from parental abuse. His mouth was covered in blood, a baseball-sized knot protruded from his forehead, another bruise formed below his eye.

"His father dropped him. Then he dropped him again."

"He dropped him twice?"

"He's been drinking."

"Where is he now?"

"Sleeping."

The baby was barely conscious, filthy diaper and a shirt that hadn't seen the laundry in weeks. Renato held him still while I secured him in the "papoose." Kids normally fight like mad when we try to restrain them, but Michael remained limp.

"Your story doesn't add up," I told the mother. She knew. Tears started.

"I have to get away from him," she said between sobs.

Michael couldn't cry. I think he was out of tears.

For the Birds

I was wondering what would possess a person who had been told earlier in the week not to take her child to an emergency room for his symptoms, which could be related to a disease-carrying bird that she had bought a week ago, then died and had been taken by the Rhode Island Department of Health for purposes I can only imagine, knowing that her two kids, herself, and her boyfriend were all ill and the home quarantined by the same Rhode Island Department of Health for more reasons I can only imagine, to call 911 because her son's flu-like symptoms were not getting better.

These thoughts occurred to me while I was standing a foot away from the ill child in a ten-by-twelve-foot bedroom with the sick mom, sick child, and the sick child's sick sister. The sick boyfriend lingered in the doorway. Joining the sick family now were four firefighters from Engine 8, who were called to the scene for a "child with difficulty breathing," myself, and Matt, my partner for the night.

"The Department of Health said not to bring him to the emergency room because they don't know what's making us sick," she said.

It was past midnight. The kid would survive, I'm sure, but I had to err on the side of caution. I put a mask over the child's nose and mouth, put him in the rescue, and took him to Hasbro Children's Hospital. The mom followed in her car.

Once at the ER, as I started to relay the information to the triage nurse, my radio interrupted the story — triple stabbing in Olneyville.

"Rescue 1 in service," I said into the mic.

"*Rescue 1, respond to Hulstead Street for a multiple stabbing, police on scene.*"

"Rescue 1, on the way."

I forgot about the dead bird and headed toward the stabbing.

CHAPTER 15
NOVEMBER

What Took So Long
A man in Cranston dies while waiting for help to arrive. His widow grieves. As days progress the questions start:

Why did it take so long for help to arrive?

Where were they?

Could he have been saved?

The answer may shock you.

Disaster strikes. 911 is called. Rescuers respond. Sometimes the problem is complex and takes dozens of emergency responders to rectify. Other times the emergency is handled by a single unit. Often, there is no emergency at all.

When is calling 911 for a medical emergency appropriate? Most folks use their best judgment before dialing. There are certain criteria: sudden pain, unusual weakness, injury, uncontrolled bleeding, unconsciousness, or any life-threatening emergency. Highly trained and properly equipped firefighters and EMTs are ready to respond at a moment's notice. Or are they?

Our society once prided ourselves on rugged individualism, fairness, and the ability to take care of ourselves and our own. The tide has turned. People now expect to be taken care of. People call 911 from their cell phones while sitting in their car so they don't have to pay for parking. They call from their homes looking for transportation, living within sight of the hospital. Doctor's offices call 911 to have noncritical patients transported to the emergency room, sometimes from the same building! Many think nothing of pushing those three buttons looking for a free ride. There is a prevailing attitude of me first, it's free, I deserve it.

Because of fear of litigation, you can call 911 for any reason and somebody will come. Nightmares. Lost dentures. Hangnails. Difficulty sleeping. Most people wouldn't dream of such irresponsible actions. Sadly, many do. And they do it often. These calls drain our resources and leave the rest of the population without adequate protection. True emergencies happen every day. Sick, dying people must wait while rescues cater to those who refuse to help themselves.

I witness the erosion of the 911 system every day. People with sore throats call 911 for a ride to the emergency room for free medical care. A person vomiting calls 911 to get free medicine. Parents of children with mild fevers call 911 so they don't have to wait, as if their problem is more important than anybody else's. Drunks call from their homes when they run out of booze, requesting detox. Kids fall and bump their head; rescues are called for ice packs.

The city of Providence is poised to reduce their firefighting force to add additional ambulances. Calls for EMS are on the rise, fires are fewer. The rationale is to move manpower from fire suppression to the rescues. What appears to be common sense is in actuality surrendering to the ideals bent on destroying our society.

Somehow, our 911 system, designed to provide highly trained and equipped personnel to the scene of an emergency, has been reduced to a glorified taxi service for those who expect to be catered to. A four-man fire company is a formidable force. Each member of the company has a vital role in every response, be it securing a water supply at a fire, doing chest compressions during CPR, or driving quickly and safely to your house when tragedy strikes. Compromising the integrity of that force to provide more rescues to a populace that abuses the system is a disservice to every responsible citizen.

Providence residents are well protected by their firefighters. You call, we come. We come with enough manpower to get the job done, no matter what that job may be. Taxpayers pay for a service and deserve to get their money's worth. It is a sad day when a proud, devastatingly effective force must be diminished to cater to a growing population that takes government services for granted, as their right, as their private taxi service.

Co-stars

"Rescue 1, respond to 356 Elmwood Avenue for an intoxicated male."

"Rescue 1, responding."

We rolled out of the bay toward our patient. Matt, my partner for the night, and I made guesses as to whom our guest might be.

"Guarantee it's Chris."

"Nope, too late."

"Kevin?"

"Nah, too far up Elmwood."

"Shingles?"

"He died last month."

"No shit?"

"Yep, died in a nursing home. Thirty-nine years old."

That quieted things down. We approached the scene slowly. There was Jimmy, weaving on the sidewalk next to a Providence police officer.

"Bitch," he said as I walked toward him.

"Cocknocker," I replied. He laughed, swore some more, and stumbled toward the rescue. On the way to the ER I told him about last night's newscast.

"Jim, we're co-stars, we were on the news last night," I said, expecting nothing but more insults.

"No shit," he said, half-smiling. "Kevin told me about it." He slurred the words but perked up. "I don't remember any of it."

No Fair

I placed the cervical collar around his neck, not because he was injured but because his neck could no longer bear the weight of his head. We put him into the stair chair as his parents looked on, hopeful, courageous, and afraid all at once.

I saw the handicapped equipment neatly arranged throughout their upstairs living space. A shower chair sat empty in a corner, leg braces leaned against a wall, next to some games. Mack understood what was going on around him but was unable to communicate with us. His eyes were slightly glazed, as they are with most postictal patients, but held my gaze with surprising intensity. I couldn't look away.

Mack's dad came with us in the rescue, leaving the boy's mother to lock up and meet us at Hasbro in the car. I had wrongly assumed Mack had cerebral palsy or something similar. I asked his dad about the boy's medical history.

"He was fine until he was five or so," he said. "Then he couldn't control his bladder. Before long he started acting up in school, nothing bad, just not paying attention, that kind of thing. Then he started falling. About a year later he started having seizures. The doctors think it might be mitochondrial disease."

I had never heard of that but if this was the result, I hope I never hear of it again.

"You have your hands full," I said to the man holding his son's hand in the back of my rescue.

Every now and then I run into somebody who I think has the courage, faith, and love to overcome anything. Mack's dad is one of these people. I think his will alone will get his boy back on his feet. For now, the boy is being treated in Boston by the best medical teams in the world.

He's nine years old. His father may never see him walk again, or even make ten.

End of the Road

"Engine 12 to fire alarm, inform Lincoln rescue that we have a code 99."

I keyed the mic.

"Rescue 1, to fire alarm, we can divert to the code."

"Roger, Rescue 1, you've got it."

Engine 12 had responded to the scene of an MVA with a possible seizure. They found a man in cardiac arrest, doors locked, car running, and its front end damaged from a collision. If everything went perfectly we could make the trip in five minutes. It took nearly ten. Buses, pedestrians, traffic, everything worked against us. Eight minutes is a long time to do CPR. I'm sure the guys from Engine 12 were listening for the sirens.

"Engine 12 to fire alarm, do you have an ETA for that rescue?"

"Rescue 1, we're at Douglas and Veazie, ETA thirty seconds."

We turned the corner at Douglas; nobody there. Sean Reddy, my partner for the day, looked around, thinking my exact thoughts. "Did we hear the right address?"

We approached Burns Street and saw the flashing lights from Engine 12. Lying on the street next to his car was our victim. Dave and Griff were doing CPR, Paul and Anthony helped with our equipment. We boarded and collared the patient and got him into the rescue, continued CPR, hooked him up to the LIFEPAK 12, started a line, analyzed the rhythm, attempted and failed to intubate. Griff got the code drugs ready, 1 epi, still asystolic. Atropine; pulseless and asystolic. More CPR. Sean drove the rescue, Anthony followed with the engine, Dave and Paul continued CPR while Griff loaded another round of epi and atropine. Possible fine V-fib, I administered a shock. Asystole, pulseless. We continued CPR up to the doorway of Roger Williams Medical Center, where the staff there took over. I gave them my report, they worked the code for at least twenty minutes while I watched, giving as much of the story as I knew.

The fifty-one-year-old man was pronounced dead at around 0900.

We cleaned and restocked the truck and were ready to go at the same time the man's widow arrived. We went back to work, she broke down in tears.

Reminiscing

Saturday night, 2100 hours. Something strange is going on—no runs for four hours. The other trucks are busy, I'm getting lucky. I had some time to sit and talk with Bob, lieutenant of Engine 14. Guys like him are invaluable to the fire department; his experience and knowledge will never be replaced.

We told some stories, his much more colorful than mine, him being from a different era, when fighting fire was the department's primary job. EMS has muscled in now, the old ways changing, and not for the better, at least from a veteran firefighter's point of view. For whatever reason, friendships were stronger then, the brotherhood a reality rather than a memory. We like to think we are different from the rest of society, and we are in a lot of ways. The nature of our work demands a certain trust in one another, our lives literally depend on us having each other's backs. We manage, enjoy the job, and make the best of it, but the present political climate and changing attitudes make it more difficult. A barrage of misleading comments from our leaders, reported by a media hungry for a story pertaining to our pay, benefits, and job performance, is wearing us down, the morale on the job at an all-time low.

Years ago, things were more simple. It was nice to forget about things for a while and talk about how things used to be.

Small World
An old friend made his way into the back of the rescue. The head umpire of the Providence Kickball League was riding his bike home when he was struck by a moving auto. I first encountered him in July on the kickball field when one of the players went down with a broken collarbone. Coincidentally, the umpire suffered the same fate as a result of the collision.

In another strange twist, I checked on the umpire after transporting an intoxicated person to the same ER. He looked up from the stretcher and asked, "Hey, aren't you the author?"

It was the first time a person I didn't know asked me that. It was a little strange. As it turns out, he works at the Brown University Bookstore and recognized me from there.

Providence seems to get smaller as the years go on.

Bookends
Thirteen hours into a thirty-eight-hour shift.
I'm not sure if my day has begun or my night has ended.
It's 0610 hours, the sun a few minutes away
Waiting to take the darkness.
In a fourth-floor apartment contractions start.
Five children, all under five years old, wake to screams.

Another is about to join them.
Her water breaks just as the sun rises.
The door is locked
The baby is born
We climb the stairs to cut the cord
And welcome a baby girl into the world.
Three hours later a grieving widow sits in a limo.
Her husband lies in his casket a few miles away.
The funeral must wait, another problem arises,
As a car crashes into the funeral procession.
She's hurt, but refuses to go.
You only bury your husband once.
We help her to the funeral home and wheel her in
Past the casket, the preacher never stops.
She sits on our stair chair,
The cervical collar digging into her skin
And listens
As her husband is laid to rest.
It's a little past noon.
One enters, one leaves.
One holds onto the miracle in her arms
As the other lets hers go.

The Times They are a Changin'
Once upon a time there were beautiful cars called Cadillacs.
People worked their entire lives so that some day they
might be able to afford one. Retired folks would take out
the machine and drive through town showing off their ride
and enjoying the day. If something were to go wrong, they
belonged to the American Automobile Association (AAA).
A simple phone call and assistance was on the way — a polite
mechanic would show up, give you a jump, change a flat, or
tow your nice Cadillac to the garage.

As years went by the Cadillac grew evil. Young men in hooded sweatshirts now "pimped" their Cadillac Escalades and rolled through the ghetto, slinging "rocks" to addicts. People feared the loathsome noise that throbbed from these shiny machines and got out of their way.

One day (today), one brave, polite mechanic in a Triple A truck had the nerve to not drive fast enough while in front of one of these machines. The driver and his friend cut off the AAA driver, pulled a gun, and beat the polite man senseless.

At least they didn't shoot him.

Doh!

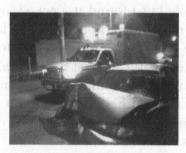

People without licenses, insurance, or registration should not drive. Especially not into trees while intoxicated.

Handful

At first she didn't like me, wouldn't listen to a word I said. She didn't want to come with us, wanted to stay right there at the shelter. The folks who run the soup kitchen thought otherwise. They had a hundred homeless people hungry for lunch and had work to do; no time to play footsies with an intoxicated thirty-seven-year-old.

I finally talked her out of the shelter and toward the rescue. She staggered and slurred but refused to let me touch her or help her walk. I kept my distance. She made it outside, where there were no walls to hold her up if should she stumble.

Once down the ramp it was nothing but us and the street, the rescue fifty feet away. I moved closer in case she started to fall.

She made a fist with her left hand and swung at me. I easily stopped the punch by holding her arm. With her right hand she grabbed my ass and gave it a good squeeze.

I don't know who laughed harder, me, her, or the crowd of homeless people watching the spectacle. We laughed all the way to the hospital. When we arrived, she sat on a stretcher and cried.

All Present and Accounted For

It took me a while but I found it, packed away in the attic, waiting for the next move, hopefully our last. It's waiting patiently on the counter in its green box for the turkey to be done, just as it has for the last fifty years, maybe more. I had to find it; things just wouldn't be the same if I used just "any" knife. It was my father's carving knife, reserved for the Thanksgiving turkey. I think of him when I carve the bird.

Ah, traditions.

Cheryl jazzed up the stuffing this year but her mom, Theresa's, signature is all over it. Her spirit follows us on holidays. It seems like yesterday the day revolved around her. Rest in peace, Mom, we miss you.

My sister Mel has my mother's china ready to be filled with traditional food. Le Sueur peas have been on a Morse table since the beginning of time. Brother Bob is home, his family together for the first time in a long, long time. I'm sure he has a relic or two left over from our parents' house. Susan is getting things ready in North Carolina, the wooden box of fine silver polished and ready to go. She doesn't change a thing from the traditional dinner, Jackie and JC wouldn't have it. We miss you, Larry—fifty are just not enough Thanksgivings.

The things we do today will live on long after we are gone. Enjoy it, it goes so fast.

Happy Thanksgiving, everybody. We're here, together on the holidays, held together by more than we realize.

Stay or Go

I had a decision to make: lock him in, or let him out. He was crouched at the rear doors of the rescue, eyes wild, screaming.

"Why you messin' with me, man!"

"Derek," I said quietly to my partner through the partition, "if he gets up, either gun it or hit the brakes, I don't care which."

Either way, JoJo would lose his balance and I would have time to throw the "net" over him. I reached over and hit the button that locks the doors just as JoJo reached for the handle.

"Why you lockin' me in, man, let me out, don't mess with me!" He glared from his position. I stayed seated in the captain's chair, portable radio loose by my side and ready for a quick draw. A portable to the noggin usually slows them down. I took the sheet from the stretcher slowly and unfolded it, ready to contain the wildman should he charge.

"If you open the door, you will fall out and the guy behind us will run you over."

JoJo stayed crouched, glaring at me. We had picked him up a few minutes ago, he and his intoxicated friend laughing and having a ball. JoJo said he wanted to go to the hospital for detox. We let him in. As soon as we got rolling he started. He unbuckled his seat belt before I could stop him, took a few steps toward me, thought better of it, then ran for the back doors and freedom. One of these days I might let one go.

I keyed the mic.

"Rescue 1 to fire alarm, advise Rhode Island we have a combative male, ETA two minutes."

We held our ground. Security took over when we arrived. Eventually JoJo was four pointed facedown on a stretcher and sedated.

Code Red!

Veazie Street, right before the second alarm. Three-and-a-half-story wood-frame residential, exposures, side one and four. The house was situated a hundred feet off Veazie at the top of a steep driveway. The narrow street left no room for mistakes with apparatus placement, and none were made. If we lost this house, there was a good chance the block would be gone in the morning.

Two firefighters from Ladder 3 climbed the aerial to the roof with a quick vent saw. Through the smoke I watched them reach the roofline, then saw them disappear as flames ripped through the fourth-floor windows. A few seconds later, when the smoke cleared, they reappeared, now at the end of the ladder, ready to get the roof.

Engine 2's pump operator nearly managed to feed a ladder pipe, three 1¾-inch attack lines and a 2½-inch master stream, before his pump cavitated, screaming for more water. He squeezed every drop from the pump but there just wasn't enough.

Engine 4 arrived at the end of Veazie, picked up another hydrant, and layed more feeders. Three hundred feet of double 3-inch feeders full of water fed their pump, and they started a relay to Engine 2. By now, Engine 5 with the air supply had arrived at the end of Veazie and pumped the hydrant, setting up a double-relay pumping operation through Engine 4 to Engine 2. With enough water to handle the demand, the pump quieted down to a hum, now efficiently doing its job as the pump operator manned the pump panel, controlling the flow of water to each individual line.

The fight raged on for three hours. I treated three firefighters for injuries, two were transported to Roger Williams Medical Center and one, after falling down a burned-out stairway, stayed working. I saw him an hour after his fall, hauling feeders. Eventually, the good guys won and the fire was extinguished. Was there ever any doubt?

Fourteen hours later, while I was home sleeping, another fire raged on the other side of the city. This one sent four firefighters to the hospital. Burns and a back injury, I'm told. Get well, brothers.

Forgotten

I used to wonder how they managed to do it. Living on the streets of Providence, hot summer days, freezing cold nights in winter, nothing more than a few layers of donated coats and maybe a blanket to keep them warm, bottle of cheap vodka giving the illusion of comfort. They have forgotten any dreams they may have once had, now they just survive each day the best they can. It's not an easy life, nor one anybody with half a brain would consider trying. The shelters show them the door early in the morning, leaving them to wander aimlessly all day, refusing entry at night if they are intoxicated, which they usually are. A few hours go by until they can scrounge up enough change to get a refill. With nowhere else to go, they call us and end up in the emergency room, not for treatment, but for survival.

I don't wonder how they do it anymore. They don't. They die. I haven't seen one hit sixty yet. Late forties, early fifties, then gone. Forgotten. A new face enters the fray as soon as there is an opening. I play along, take them to the hospital, and watch them die. Sometimes it takes years.

Hmm . . .

Chest pain in a holding cell is a difficult call. All instinct leads you to believe it's a case of cellitis, and it usually is. The hospital beats the prison, most times. When the patient is your own age skepticism is overwhelming. When it is the second time you have been called to the same holding cell in two hours, it's guaranteed.

Sometimes.

Veronica sat on the steel bench, crying. She was in desperate need of a shower and some new clothes. I asked how she was feeling.

"I've had pain in my chest since last night but didn't say anything," she said quietly.

Hmm. Usually the theatrics could win an Academy Award. We put her on the stretcher and rolled her out of the cell. I asked the sherriff for the paperwork, he said there was none, she was free to go home. Double hmm. I asked her to rate the pain on a one-to-ten scale.

"It's about a seven now but last night it was around four." Triple hmm. Fakers rate a guaranteed ten.

Once in the rescue we did some vitals and ran a 12 lead EKG. BP was 180/120, heart rate 110, SpO_2 91 percent. The EKG was abnormal with a right bundle branch block. She had a history of an irregular heartbeat but couldn't afford her medications. We started her on O_2, gave her some aspirin and a nitro, and started toward Rhode Island Hospital. On the way her phone rang. Her mother was home with her grandchildren waiting for her daughter to come home.

"Mama, don't cry, I'll be home soon," Veronica said into the phone, then started crying herself.

I have no idea why she was detained and didn't ask. Not because I wasn't curious, I was, I just didn't feel it was any of my business. I can only wonder why a nice lady the same age as me with a family who cared deeply about her was in jail.

Her birthday was five days after mine; we shared this earth for nearly exactly the same amount of time. Is it fate, bad choices, or circumstance that put us on such opposite paths? I can only wonder.

CHAPTER 16
DECEMBER

Resurrection
I asked him his name. He spelled it out.
    "A-r-o-u-a-r-t-i-o-u-n."
    "How do you pronounce it?"
    "Arouartioun."
    "Is that Armenian?"
    "Yes, it means Resurrection."
    "What's your date of birth?"
    "December 24, 1935."
    "Hence, the Resurrection."
He shrugged and smiled, his abdominal pain that made
him call 911 gone for now, no particular reason. He said the
pain has been coming and going for two weeks, no idea why.
Perhaps today they would find the answer. We had a nice
talk on the way to the ER. His family moved from Armenia
following the genocide of 1915 to Syria, where he grew up.
    "Nice place, Syria, they gave us land, said to stay there."
Refugees were given a chance to rebuild their lives. Some
went to Europe, some the Middle East, some America. His
family moved back to Armenia in the fifties when it was part
of the Soviet Union.
    "We were very poor. My father retired from the French
Army in 1946, not much of a pension then."

Somehow they managed to escape from Soviet Russia; his wife had family in America. They have a nice home in the Reservoir Triangle area of Providence now, grandchildren, maybe a great-grandchild on the way. We arrived at the hospital, Arouartioun insisted on walking in.

I couldn't help being inspired by his story. I'll be moving, again, in a couple of weeks, three streets away from the house I've been renting for six months. It looks like I've finally found a home. I didn't have to travel the world to find it.

CHAPTER 17
JANUARY

Maniac

January 1, 0200 hours. We turned the corner into mayhem. A car sped toward a group of people, striking one, throwing him onto the hood then onto the street. Others first ran toward the victim, then saw the car do a 180-degree turn and fishtail back toward the victim. People scattered every which way, the enraged driver went for the guy lying in the street. He miraculously avoided being hit a second time.

Veakro stopped the rescue in front of the victim, put on the lights, and stepped out while I radioed for police. Unbelievably, the car did another 180 and buzzed the rescue. The guy on the street managed to stand and walk toward the sidewalk, right before the car made another pass.

Somehow, nobody was killed. As the maniac sped toward the city we treated the victim and tried to calm the crowd. They had been out for the evening, rented a limousine which overheated on the highway. They stopped at an adult entertainment nightclub on Allens Avenue because one of the passengers knew a bouncer there and they wanted to use the restroom. The limo driver told me later that this was her first nighttime job. She heard the money was terrific.

"I'm going back to taking people to the airport," she said, still shaking from witnessing the madness.

The cops came a few minutes later and took a report.
New Year's Eve 2007 was over. A new year had begun.

Rash of Stabbings
I've had a few days off since the New Year's Eve Massacre.
(Stabbings, assaults, pedestrian struck, man out a window,
head lacerations, concussions, and a nineteen-year-old who
eventually delivered the state's first baby of the new year.)

Add another stabbing to a recent rash of stabbings here in
the capital city. A deliveryman was attacked by four men as
he sat outside Stop & Shop in the Manton neighborhood. They
beat and robbed him, eventually stabbing him in the stomach.
Last week three young men were stabbed during an incident
near Broad Street. My patient was a nineteen-year-old with
three wounds to his upper torso. Whoever did the stabbing
was not kidding around; he was going for a kill. The last
call of the night on New Year's Eve was for a man with stab
wounds sitting on a porch near Thurbers Avenue. I found five
stab wounds on this guy, one of which punctured a lung. As
I walked out of the trauma room at Rhode Island Hospital,
another man walked into the ER holding his intestines in his
hands. He was attacked on the same block as my patient.

I wonder if all of this is coincidence or if there's a slasher
in our midst.

Madison's Class

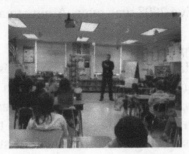

I had the pleasure of visiting my cousin Madison's third-grade classroom recently. She wanted me to talk about my experience as an author but her classmates seemed more interested in my experience as a firefighter. I only put a few of the kids to sleep; the rest tolerated my story and treated me well.

Thank you, Madison, Mrs. Raver, and the rest of the class for the opportunity to speak to you and answer your questions. (Even the one about stealing the man in the wheelchair's boots!) I had a lot of fun.

Dehydrated

"Why did you call 911?"

"I'm dehydrated."

"You don't look dehydrated."

"What do dehydrated people look like?"

"Get in the truck."

He stood outside the Providence Rescue Mission, smoking a cigarette. He wore his forty years badly; I would have sworn he was sixty. He stepped into the rescue and made himself comfortable on the bench seat as I started my report.

"How long have you been dehydrated?"

"Since last night."

"Really."

"Yup. A water line broke and I don't have running water."

"When did the line break?"

"Last night."

I closed my eyes and started counting.

"One thousand one, one thousand two, one thousand three . . ."

Lips

"What's the matter?" I asked John, who stood outside of a Dunkin' Donuts sipping a coffee.

"My lips are bleeding."

"No they're not."

He bit his bottom lip hard enough to produce a few droplets.

"I have AIDS."

"Really."

"Full blown."

"Get in the truck."

I took him to the ER. He had just left. I was there last night at midnight when another Providence rescue brought him in, reason unknown.

All of the psych beds in the state are full, the chest pain unit at Rhode Island Hospital now being used as a holding area. I have no idea where to bring the next one.

Turning the Corner

He usually called from a pay phone on Broad Street. It seemed strange seeing him in his home. The front steps looked weak; I tested them with my foot before putting my full weight on each tread. The "Beware of Dog" sign was a nice shot of self-esteem for the fifty-year-old mutt who lay chained to the inside stairs. He put a halfhearted growl out there for anybody interested. For his sake I stepped to the other side of the entryway as we walked past.

Too bad it never rains inside I thought as we walked through a few rooms into a rear bedroom. This place could have used a rinse. It hadn't seen the business end of a vacuum or broom in decades. Filth festers when it has nowhere to go.

Our patient lay on a couch, seizing. His vacant stare looked past us at something only he could see, his body shaking and rigid. It was a mild seizure and only lasted a few seconds. The shaking managed to loosen an empty pint of vodka from the filthy cushions.

"He didn't take his meds," said a dark lady who suddenly popped out of a doorway. "Said he'd drink a corner and be all right."

We loaded him onto the stair chair and into the bright sunshine, careful not to fall through the porch steps. He seized again when we got him into the truck. When he came out of it I asked him how much he had to drink.

"A corner."

I thought back to the empty vodka bottle and envisioned an inch of booze at the bottom, when tipped to drink, filling the "corner" of the bottle.

We took him around the corner to Rhode Island Hospital.

Comfort One
The Comfort One protocol spares terminal patients the indignity, pain, and discomfort of life-saving efforts by EMS personnel. Patients can opt for comfort measures only during their last days or hours. No CPR, no intubation, no IVs for cardiac drugs. Basically we provide oxygen and comfort.

Our patient wore such a bracelet. His two-year battle with cancer appeared to be nearing an end. He started having trouble breathing yesterday, followed by muscle cramping. I have taken him to the hospital numerous times in the past and was inspired by his and his family's courage. It was sad to see it come to this. Henry carried him down the snow-covered stairs of the second-floor apartment that will be his final home and into the rescue. He never complained.

We gave him supplemental oxygen and brought him to the hospital.

Hasbro Children's Hospital.

He's eight years old.

Sacrificing the Body

The steps were wide, perhaps six feet across. An inch of snow covered the treads; I saw footprints lead to our patient, a forty-five-year-old female.

"I've got two witnesses," was the first thing she said, followed by, "I told the landlord to take care of these steps. He don't do nothin' but take money."

"Can you move?" I asked.

"No."

"Can you wiggle your toes?"

"No."

"Can you feel your legs?"

"No."

Great.

Ladder Company 5's crew managed to get her onto the longboard and stretcher. I asked one of the "witnesses" what happened.

"She fell down the stairs."

I looked at the six steps. The footprints went directly to the indentation in the snow where we found the patient. The snow on the steps was uninterrupted other than the footprints.

I grabbed the bottom of the stretcher and lifted my end. The three hundred–pound woman felt like six as the stretcher, and my back, groaned under her weight. Her cell phone rang, she answered, told the person on the other end to "talk to the paramedic, I'm being rushed to the hospital," and handed it to me.

"I thought you couldn't move?" I said.

The folks at Rhode Island Hospital knew her name before I said it. She's a weekly visitor. Nothing like sacrificing the body to keep our citizens safe. Or, in her case, to make a little money.

Tough Guy

Lunchtime, one of my favorite times of day. I had made stuffed meatloaf, always a favorite with the guys. Wayne called them meat bombs, which I guess they were. A big ball of hamburger, a couple of eggs, secret seasonings, separated into twelve "bombs," sliced down the middle, add some spinach and cheddar, an hour at 350 and presto!

Two bites in the bell tipped.

"Engine 2 with Rescue 3, respond to the corner of North Main and Doyle for a pedestrian struck."

We dropped our forks and hit the pole. I was looking forward to getting back to lunch. I drove the engine, looking ahead, fully confident that whatever happened at North Main and Doyle we would handle and be back before the food got cold.

In the distance I saw what looked to be a bundle of bloody rags, tiny. Further up the road, about a hundred yards away, was a bigger bundle. I stopped the truck and stepped out. What looked like a woman was lying on her back, her legs somehow straddling her head. A human body was not meant to be crushed by the wheels of a tractor trailer. She was conscious and hysterical.

"The baby!" she said.

I saw an off-duty Providence firefighter in the distance pick up the bundle and start CPR. Rescue 3 had arrived and was treating the woman, another rescue was called for the other victim.

Parts of a mangled stroller covered the hundred yards between the woman and the other "bundle of rags." The eighteen-wheel semi was stopped in the middle of the road, a little further up. Somehow, I helped the crew from Rescue 3 immobilize the woman and get her into the rescue. Her legs and back were broken, probably paralyzed. There is no training for what we encountered, you just make do.

Rescue 5 arrived; I joined them in the back of their rescue. Okie, the off-duty firefighter, blood covering his face, handed the infant to Greg and Kevin. The baby was dead. We continued CPR, tried to start a line and get a tube, and sped toward the ER.

The snow-covered sidewalk on the corner of North Main and Doyle made it impossible to pass. The woman—the baby's grandmother I found out later—was forced to use the street just as the truck was making the turn. The driver never saw them. The baby carriage was caught between the rear wheels and dragged down North Main Street. The grandmother's lower torso was crushed by the wheels. She stayed put until we arrived.

Somehow, the grandmother survived the ordeal. The baby never had a chance.

An hour later we returned to our meatloaf. It was silent in the day room as we ate. Engine 2 was called back to the scene for a "wash down." Chief Ronny Moura, wise from twenty-five years of experience, called us off and sent another engine company to wash the blood from the city street.

I remember thinking that I had to eat, even though it was the last thing I wanted to do. I was new to the job then, wanted to look tough.

Big tough guy sixteen years later, I remember it like it was yesterday.

Little Man

The little man Henry carried through the snow last month passed away last night. His two-year battle with cancer has come to an end. His mom and twin brother must be heartbroken. I remember going to their apartment at all hours of the night when the boy needed help, watching his mom run around the apartment while we put her son on the stair chair, gathering last-minute things for the trip to the hospital while a healthy version of the patient looked on, never complaining, just watching, as if the drama that unfolded in front of him wasn't real. He never said a word, just helped his mother and came along.

I imagine the little family will heal, and move on, no longer needing us. It's too bad they needed us in the first place.

Rest in peace, brother.

Different Worlds

The baby was still, staring blankly at nothing. This had happened before, only not for as long. After a minute the parents called 911. Two more minutes before the first help arrived. The guys from Engine 4 entered the home just as the baby came out of his seizure. We were still five minutes away, responding from the other end of Providence.

The East Side is different from South Providence. The streets are tree lined and quiet, a fire truck causes quite a commotion. I don't think we are even noticed on the other side, our trips into the neighborhood commonplace.

"Engine 4 to Rescue 1, we have an eighteen-month-old male, conscious and alert at this time following three minutes of seizure activity. History of febrile seizures."

"*Rescue 1, received.*"

I put the mic back into the cradle as Rob, my new partner, turned onto North Main. Two minutes later we joined Engine

4 and the patient. Neighbors looked out windows and filled doorways, concerned. Bob Randle, the officer of Engine 4, met me outside and gave the preliminary report. The baby was in the doorway of his home, held by his dad as his mother sat in a chair in the living room holding an infant. An old dog came over, sniffed my leg, decided I was okay, and went back to the couch, satisfied there was no danger here.

The baby was fine. The parents had the proper medication to treat the situation and decided to take care of it themselves. They apologized for "bothering" us. We talked for a while, insisted they call for help whenever they felt it necessary, no bother whatsoever, this is our job. They stood in the doorway and waved as we drove away.

Sometimes I think a spaceship picked me up and put me on another planet. Then I remember, this is how it's supposed to be.

Miscommunication

"Overweight, history of hypertension, chest pain, history of heart attack, diaphoretic . . ." He counted off the risk signs on his fingers while shaking his head.

A few minutes prior I had brought an overweight, sweat-covered fiftyish man to the ER. Ron took one look at the guy, quickly read my report, and put him into a critical care room.

"Why is he here?" asked the doctor on call impatiently, annoyed that we brought the patient to critical care.

"Look at him," replied Ron as Rob and I transferred the patient from our stretcher to theirs.

"He needs an EKG," said the doctor.

"We'll do it here, this is where he belongs," said Ron.

The doctor shook his head and walked away.

The critical care team got to work, IVs started, leads placed, oxygen administered.

We had already done an EKG prior to nitro and aspirin, I handed the results to the doctor when he returned. He put the paper aside without a second glance. I wasn't surprised.

"Is that guy an idiot?" I asked Ron, referring to the doctor in the critical care room when I left the trauma room and returned to the triage desk.

"I believe he is," replied Ron, who immediately shifted gears and took a report from the next crew that had arrived.

The patient's nephew stood nearby, listening. A few minutes later the charge nurse approached Ron and told him that the patient's family had filed a complaint against him, and maybe me. I'll find out in a few days. He didn't like the way we were talking about his uncle.

You would think he had more important things to worry about.

Lord of the Rings

"I know, I'll put five key rings around my penis just to see what happens. Nothing yet, maybe I'll thumb through the recent Penthouse *to see what happens. Uh-oh, didn't see this coming, better call 911 and have them take a look."*

Security

We are all in this field for similar reasons. Saving lives, helping the sick and injured, making money, gaining self-respect, and the camaraderie are all part of the bigger picture. The people I work with in the local emergency rooms are just as dedicated as the firefighters I live with.

A group of people that seldom, if ever, get mentioned or praise is the security guards. These men and women are vital to the successful operation of the ER, especially those at Rhode Island Hospital. Just today a guard named John, a big, quiet guy from the South Providence neighborhood, helped get a patient who refused to leave the back of the rescue into the ER. I never asked, just informed him that I was bringing him a combative patient. He took it upon himself to help us out. Another guard, Amir, also from South Providence, helped a Spanish-speaking patient communicate with the nurse trying to figure out what was ailing her. I'm sure no compensation is involved for the extra work and it would be just as easy to walk away, but Amir and most of his peers are willing to help when needed.

I've seen these people respectfully restrain the most violent, abusive patients in a calm, professional manner, never losing their cool while taking some obscene abuse from those they are helping. Black guards are routinely called niggers by drunken fools, the female guards endure their own share of harassment.

They somehow manage to turn the other cheek and do a great job.

A lot of pieces have to come together for things to work, lives to be saved, and safety ensured. These folks are a bigger part of the puzzle than most people realize.

Overdose
"Engine 3 to Rescue 1, unconscious male, looks like a heroin overdose."

"Rescue 1, received."

Rob stopped the rescue in front of the building and got out. I grabbed the blue bag from the side compartment; Rob went to the rear doors and pulled the stretcher from the rig. I placed the bag full of drugs and supplies on top of the stretcher and we made our way in. A man held the door for us, informing us that the elevators were out of order. We left the stretcher at the bottom of the stairs and made our way up.

A man in his fifties lay on his back, shallow respirations, normal pulse with a bluish tint to his skin.

"He's been down for about ten minutes," said Joe, Engine 3's officer. "Went to the bathroom and didn't come out. His friends went in to get him, this is how they found him."

The clear plastic of the non-rebreather clouded up every eight seconds or so, the reservoir of pure oxygen barely dented.

"Rob, get the trauma board." I said. I hoped the Narcan would be effective and we wouldn't need it. "Better get a bag ready."

Another Joe from Engine 3 prepared an IV as I drew up 2 mg of Narcan. Instead of waiting for a line I administered the drug into the dying man's triceps. Instead of the patient improving, he stopped breathing completely.

We had the man intubated and the first round of epi on board just as Rob returned with the board. We secured all two hundred pounds of him, ventilated, and got ready for descent. Everybody on scene pitched in every way possible getting him down the stairs and into the rescue. We brought him to the Rhode Island Hospital ER, where the trauma team took over. Half an hour later they called it.

Time of death: 1836 hours. Engine 3 headed back to the barn, Rob put the truck together, and I tried to make sense of the paperwork. A man is dead, I barely blinked and it was back to business as usual. Sometimes I think this job takes more than it gives.

Party

She sat on the step of Engine 8, her dress ripped, no coat, shivering in the wind and snow. A one-inch laceration to the top of her head and a huge welt on her left temple, evidence of an assault. Blood streamed down her face, ruining the makeup she must have spent a long time applying. I imagine she spent hours getting ready for a fun night on the town.

Somebody cracked her head with a bottle. The bars had just let out, spilling hundreds of drunken revelers into the streets of Providence. The chest pains, seizures, and breathing difficulties would continue to trickle in but for the next hour or two our rescues will be tied up with assaults, robberies, and other assorted mayhem. Witnessing the aftermath of a night on the town makes me wonder why people even bother to go out.

Emergency Response for the Mentally Ill

The blinds separated, leaving an inch of blackness between them. Somewhere in the darkness two eyes peered out. They saw me; I couldn't see them.

"Rescue 1 to fire alarm, do you have a callback number?"

"Stand by."

We stood on the snow-covered doorstep. No sounds came from inside. I knocked again. Nothing.

My portable radio cracked the silence. *"Rescue 1?"*

"Go ahead."

"The person should be opening the door, I've got her on the phone."

"Roger, the door is opening."

A disheveled, intoxicated thirty-year-old female opened the door widely, begging us to come in and shut the door. The place was in shambles. Dirty dishes, laundry, spent cigarette butts, animal waste, and cockroaches had taken over. The patient scurried about, pretending to tidy up the place but in actuality couldn't have tied her shoes at this point, she was too far gone.

"Rescue 1, do you need the police?" the radio blared.

"No police!" screamed the patient. "I'm sick, not a criminal!"

And so it goes.

The fire department is called for a variety of reasons. Nestled among the building fires, chest pain, intoxicated persons, building collapses, car accidents, and other emergencies are a surprising number of calls for psychologically unstable patients. The labels vary — emotional, change of mental status, anxious, suicidal — but all are potentially dangerous.

Society is filled with people suffering from emotional and psychological problems. Many of these folks lead productive lives once helped by remarkably effective treatments; therapy and medication produce tangible results in the mentally ill. Some patients have given up on treatment, choosing to make their own way in the world unimpeded by modern medicine. Most are not successful. Many have no access to the health care system. Whether that is their own decision or beyond their control is irrelevant; what matters is there are a lot of untreated mentally ill people living among us.

When crisis occurs, and if they are able to recognize the warning signals their damaged minds send out, a good resource is the 911 system. Highly trained personnel are waiting to take care of these patients, get them the help they so desperately need.

Or are they?

Those in the field of EMS are given rudimentary training regarding the mentally ill. They cannot solve their problems, nor do they have the qualifications to try. The best they can do is to keep the patient calm and get them to the help they so desperately need. Sound simple? It's not.

When a person decides to call for help, they are at the end of a long, downward spiral. Making that cry for help is a courageous step, fraught with uncertainty. They wait by the phone, wondering if they did the right thing by calling. From the time the initial call is made to the time help arrives a lot can happen. They change their mind. They hear voices. They begin to see their rescuers as threats to their independence.

At times violent struggles ensue. Sometimes the situation is defused with care and compassion; often, force must be used. But whose responsibility is it to use force?

The majority of calls for help in Providence concerning the mentally ill are handled by the fire department EMS, not the police. Family members and friends who call want to avoid a confrontation. They are at the end of their rope, helpless and afraid. They look to EMS as saviors when they arrive to take their loved one to a hospital or psychiatric facility, only to find their options limited by law and lack of training.

Patients who make the call of their own accord don't see themselves as a threat. What lucidity remained when they called for help is often gone when help arrives. These emotionally charged situations often lead to violent confrontations with would-be rescuers.

Mental health care professionals call 911 from their facilities looking for an ambulance to take a problem patient off their hands. EMTs are then expected to put that volatile patient into a four by eight–foot space filled with glass and needles. It is a recipe for disaster.

EMS professionals cannot restrain, subdue, or abduct. Doing so is a violation of a person's civil rights. There are no men in the white coats. We do not carry straitjackets. All we have is common sense, compassion, and a willingness to help a person in need. Often, it is not enough.

In the tragic aftermath of one such recent call in Pawtucket, a mentally ill man was shot and killed. The police solved the crisis the only way they could at the time. The officer justifiably felt his life in danger and responded accordingly. Would the result have been different if the fire department had been called, or would there be a dead EMT in the patient's place? We will never know.

A rapid intervention team consisting of a psychiatrist with power to commit a patient, a law enforcement officer with power to restrain a person against their will, and a pair of EMTs to provide support and transportation in a safe environment is what is needed on these type of calls. Until that happens, we are sending undertrained, unarmed, and overwhelmed people into dangerous situations. There needs to be a definitive approach to handling the mentally ill who call for help. The current system is a time bomb. You can hear it ticking if you care to listen.

"No police," I said as softly as possible. "Get your things and come with us. We'll get you some help." I looked around for potential weapons, kitchen knives especially. A caseworker was stabbed in the neck on Broad Street a few years ago by an emotional patient, bled to death in the doorway, leaving a wife and two small children.

After fifteen minutes of negotiations, crying, laughing, and a temper tantrum or two, we left the woman's apartment, from the looks of things for a long time.

Good Day

"Rescue 1 and Engine 13, respond to 328 Calla Street for an infant not breathing."

Seconds seem like hours. Cars move like dinosaurs on the brink of extinction, sirens and lights ineffective. Gloves go on, mind racing, ghosts invade, I throw them out, the trucks move faster, picking up speed, three minutes pass. Before we stop I'm out the door, mother running, baby in her arms, blue. I take her; she's stiff, burning with fever, rigid, then starts to seize.

Oxygen, assisted ventilations, family screaming, everybody tries to do something, I give out tasks, an IV, keep bagging, need a glucose test, find the history, learn Spanish quickly, I need to know what's going on, get a temp, find out her weight, find a pulse, keep her safe, the seizing continues as if she were possessed.

Pulsox rises, seizing continues, can't get an IV, family hysterical, firefighters busy now, doing their job, Tylenol suppository administered, temp of 104, need a driver, call the hospital, tell them we're coming in with an eighteen-month-old, possible febrile seizure, ETA one minute.

Give the crowd that has gathered a thumbs-up, look calm, reassuring I hope, close the door and take the mother's hand, seat her next to the stretcher, let her know it will be okay, seizing slows down, the baby relaxes a little, the truck rolls, calm now, all we can do is done.

Trauma room ready, medical team takes over, struggle for a while with the IV but eventually get one, Broselow tape extended, dosages and medication ordered, bagging continues.

We clean and restock the truck, another child is having a seizure at school, have to go. Twenty minutes, we're back, no seizure, just a kid who took a ball to the face, iced him down, brought him in and checked on the baby who wasn't breathing, she's breathing on her own now, fever down, still bluish but okay, mother cries and hugs me.

Yeah, it's a good day.

Brittany
I'm dog tired and look it. I can feel the bags under my eyes dragging my face to the pavement. People pass, I barely look at them, just enough to avoid contact. I'm isolated, lost in my thoughts, just trying to make it home.

A pizza I ordered waits for me at Pizza Pier. I can see the storefront in the distance, a few hundred feet away. I walk past the sushi restaurant that shares the same block, peek in the window as I pass, and notice a beautiful young girl sitting at one of the tables that line the outside windows. It's just a glance, a fraction of a second, but I feel a little better.

I'm waiting for my pizza. Marlin, the guy behind the counter, is busy with somebody else. I wait, and slouch a little, the hours having finally caught up with me. Thirty-four hours since my last encounter with unconsciousness. It's different being a civilian in Providence, the uniform gone, the radio on somebody else's belt and the crushing weight of being on duty lifted, for now.

"Michael." (It's okay she calls me Michael, I met her when she was four.)

I turn and there is the beautiful young girl standing next to me. I'm filled with such ridiculous happiness I can't believe how good I feel.

"You look tired," she says, and gives me a hug.

"Just a little."

We talk a little, hope to get together this weekend. I want to join her and her friend but I just don't have the gas, and it would be a little tacky to bring a pizza into a sushi place, I think. I pay for the pizza and we walk out together. We say good-bye, and she leaves me, to join her friend back at the table by the window. I look in again as I walk past, smile and wave to them.

I don't feel so alone when I get back to my car, turn the key, and head away from the city toward home. I'm not as tired, either. I feel good. Great actually, and savor every second of happiness that an unexpected encounter with my daughter has given to me.

AFTERWORD

Who am I to be witness to such human tragedy, triumph, and tedium? Why has my journey led me to other people's emergencies? Why do I love it so?

I honestly do not know. I have been present at the end of a person's struggle for life, watched as their final breath left their body and all I could do to keep it going was not enough; been there at the beginning, holding a newborn whose first breath came in the back of an ambulance in the middle of the night; and in the middle, when the weight of despair and disillusionment became too much, and the muzzle of a gun ended up in the mouth, sweaty finger on the trigger, body still warm, heart no longer beating.

It is a very private world that I am invited into day after day and night after night. People's worst moments are shared with me, and they look to me for salvation, or at least a way to get them there. I do what I can, help them breathe, stop their bleeding, stop their seizing, and make them feel better. Or at least try.

Thank you for reading. And if you ever needed me, thank you for the opportunity.

ABOUT THE AUTHOR

Michael Morse spent twenty-three years working in Providence, Rhode Island as a firefighter/EMT before retiring in 2013 as Captain, Rescue Co. 5. His books and articles offer fellow firefighters, EMT's and the general population alike a poignant glimpse into one person's journey through his life and work.

Morse lives in Warwick, Rhode Island with his wife, Cheryl, two Maine Coon cats, Lunabelle and Victoria Mae and Mr. Wilson, their dog. They have two daughters, Danielle and Brittany.